CREDIT CRUNCH HEALTH CARE

How economics can save our publicly funded health services

Cam Donaldson

First published in Great Britain in 2011 by

The Policy Press
University of Bristol
Fourth Floor
Beacon House
Queen's Road
Bristol BS8 1QU
UK
t: +44 (0)117 331 4054
f: +44 (0)117 331 4093
tpp-info@bristol.ac.uk
www.policypress.co.uk

North American office:
The Policy Press
c/o International Specialized Books Services
920 NE 58th Avenue, Suite 300
Portland, OR 97213-3786, USA
t: +1 503 287 3093
f: +1 503 280 8832
info@isbs.com

British Library Cataloguing in Publication Data
A catalogue record for this book is available from the British Library.

Library of Congress Cataloging-in-Publication Data
A catalog record for this book has been requested.

ISBN 978 1 84742 752 6 paperback
ISBN 978 1 84742 753 3 hardcover

Cover design by Qube Design Associates, Bristol
Front cover: photograph kindly supplied by iStockphoto.
Printed and bound in Great Britain by Hobbs, Southampton

For one woman who helped me with my homework
and another who is a Scottish internationalist at talking

Contents

List of figures, tables and boxes

Figures

Tables

Boxes

About the author

Cam Donaldson holds the Yunus Chair in Social Business and Health at Glasgow Caledonian University. From 2002-10, he held the Health Foundation Chair in Health Economics at Newcastle University, where he was founding director of the Institute of Health and Society and professor in the Newcastle University Business School. He held the Svare Chair in Health Economics at the University of Calgary from 1998-2002, having first become a professor of health economics in 1996 while at the Health Economics Research Unit at the University of Aberdeen.

Cam has received numerous competitive awards in recognition of his research, having been:

- an inaugural National Institute for Health Research Senior Investigator (2008-12);
- a Public Services Fellow in the Advanced Institute for Management Research (2004-05), funded by the UK's Economic and Social Research Council;
- a Canadian Institutes for Health Research Senior Investigator (2000-02); and
- a Senior Scholar (1998-2003), funded by the Alberta Heritage Foundation for Medical Research.

Over the past 25 years, Cam has published over 200 peer-reviewed articles in economics, medical, health policy and health management journals and has co-authored or edited several books on various aspects of health economics and public service delivery.

This book is a little different to Cam's previous outputs. It is not aimed at a specialist academic audience. Rather, it seeks to persuade a more general audience of health care professionals and the public about the importance of economics in explaining why we have the types of health care systems we have and how we can make these systems better serve the public by improving our understanding of the economic notion of 'value' and how it can be utilised in managing our limited, but valuable, health care resources.

Not many are better placed to do this because of the extensive links and collaborations Cam has fostered with clinicians and managers at all levels of health care systems internationally during his 25 years in health economics research.

Acknowledgements

There are many people to whom I am eternally grateful for giving me the confidence, encouragement and ability to write this book.

I was given a good start in health economics, by mentors such as Alan Maynard (York), John Forbes (Glasgow, now Edinburgh), Ian Russell and John Bond (Newcastle) and Gavin Mooney (Aberdeen). Senga Bond, also of Newcastle, has always believed in me and given me the confidence to do stuff differently. In my early days at York, I shared an office with Steve Birch, now at McMaster University in Ontario, who has been great friend and critic over the past 25 years.

As many of my colleagues know, I love working in teams. In this way, I have worked with many great people over the years, and the ones who will recognise some of the material in the book are Rachel Baker, Angela Bate, Stirling Bryan, Gillian Currie, Karen Gerard, Dorte Eyrd-Hansen, Steve Jan, Mike Jones-Lee, Graham Loomes, Braden Manns, Helen Mason, Craig Mitton, Jan Abel Olsen, Stuart Peacock, Jose-Luis Pinto Prades, Jim Rankin, Angela Robinson, Danny Ruta, Mandy Ryan, Phil Shackley, Alan Shiell and Virginia Wiseman.

I would also like to thank our dear friends Jim and Miggie Rankin, Gillian Currie and Mark Cassano, and Tom Noseworthy and colleagues in the Department of Community Health Sciences at the University of Calgary and the Alberta Children's Hospital. Likewise, Stirling Bryan and Anne Backhouse, and Craig Mitton and Michelle Jenkins. All hosted me in one way or other during summer 2009 when I wrote most of this book. Jim and Craig also read drafts, and I am most grateful for the comments received. I have learned so much about health care from Jim Rankin, a professor of nursing at the University of Calgary.

I have also received tremendous encouragement over the years and in the writing of this book from three leading clinicians. Alastair Noble would describe himself as a general practitioner from Nairn, but is much more than that. Occasionally in the book, I use the phrase 'a clinical decision is a purchasing decision'. This masterly statement is attributable to Alastair. Whenever I talk to Sir Muir Gray, one of the all-time leading lights of public health, the first question he always asks is, "What are you writing, Cam?" He was particularly positive about my plans for this book. Sir Michael Rawlins got me involved at the National Institute for Health and Clinical Excellence and has welcomed me as part of the 'NICE family' ever since. He has done an enormous amount for many aspects of health and health care policy, and not least health economics. I am deeply honoured to have him write the foreword to this book.

Until moving to Glasgow Caledonian, my previous eight years of funding came from the Health Foundation. I am deeply indebted to the Foundation for this support, to the National Institute for Health Research for its recognition of my work and to Newcastle University for employing me as Health Foundation Chair in Health Economics from 2002–10.

Finally, I cannot thank my family enough for the love and support they have given me over the years, permitting me to accumulate the experience to allow me to write this piece. Diane, Graham, Callum and Dominic – love you guys, always.

Foreword

Thirty years ago, those interested in the economics of health and health care were confined to the groves of academia. Snubbed by general economists, health economists were regarded as little more than upstarts with nothing relevant or interesting to say. And they were regarded by clinicians as unnecessary and irrelevant. How the world has changed.

Every country in the world is facing demands for increased expenditure at a time when resources are finite. Every country is seeking to restrain health care expenditure as the prices of new technologies – many with significant advantages – are increasing year on year. Clinicians can no longer ignore the economic cost of providing for all the health care needs of their patients. As the late (and very great) Sir George Godber – Chief Medical Officer of England from 1960 to 1973 – once famously said, "When a doctor sees a patient in his consulting room he must also remember those in the waiting room."

In this book Cam Donaldson provides an insight into the economics of health care that is accessible to non-experts including clinicians. He starts with a critical examination of some of the diverse approaches that developed countries have taken to financing health care, public versus private provision and the impact of charges. He pays considerable attention to 'programme budgeting and marginal analysis' as well as to formal methods of economic evaluation including the quality adjusted life year measure. All this with hardly a single mathematical formula.

This book will appeal to those lacking any formal training in health economics. I commend it, particularly, to those like me who can hardly understand their bank statements let alone their income tax forms. And for tomorrow's health professionals, it is a must. They are going to struggle, throughout their professional lives, if they cannot get to grips with the realities of the modern world.

Sir Michael Rawlins
London, June 2010

ONE

Introduction: the quid pro quo of health care

The market is coming. Despite the gross and widespread failure of markets to deliver on societies' needs in recent years, the ironic consequence will be the reduced ability of governments to invest in public services. Governments are already spending public money in new ways, shoring up the banks and other parts of the private sector. This will lead to a claimed lack of ability to keep health services public, and the perfect opportunity for advocates of market forces and deregulation in health care to pounce. A gradual privatisation of health care has been taking place in some major economies of the world already. This is illustrated in Table 1.1. Although for 14 of 27 countries listed in the table the proportion of health care expenditures coming from the public purse has either been maintained or has increased over a period of almost 20 years, for the most advanced economies in this group, any increases are slight. As ever, the US is an exception, as its public sector contribution to health care funding continues to grow significantly. The point is that the pattern is not clear cut and in other advanced economies such as Canada and Sweden decreases in the share of spending coming from the public purse have been quite significant – and this has been during the good times. The opportunity is now here for more radical change in terms of pushing the agenda for greater private financing of health care. Some governments will be convinced, and make no mistake – if they could dispose of their obligations to health care financing on the basis that it could be more efficiently financed through other means, they would.

More than ever, therefore, it is important to make the case for public financing of our health services. However, we need to make that case on the same grounds as the market reformers – that of efficiency as well as equity. But, there is a quid pro quo. Strictly, in

Table 1.1: Total health expenditure, and percentage of total that is public, in OECD countries (1990 and 2006)

Country	1990 total health expenditure, US$PPP	% public	2006 total health expenditure, US$PPP	% public	Absolute % increase
Australia	1,318	67	3,141	68	+1
Austria	1,205	74	3,606	76	+2
Canada	1,678	75	3,678	70	−5
Czech Rep	576	96	1,509	88	−8
Denmark	1,453	83	3,362	84	+1
Finland	1,292	81	2,668	76	−5
France	1,520	78	3,449	80	+2
Germany	1,602	76	3,371	77	+1
Greece	707	63	2,483	62	−1
Iceland	1,376	87	3,340	82	−5
Ireland	796	72	3,082	78	+6
Italy	1,321	78	2,614	77	−1
Japan	1,082	78	2,578	81	+3
South Korea	371	37	1,464	55	+18
Luxembourg	1,486	93	4,303	91	−2
Mexico	260	41	792	44	+3
Netherlands	1,403	78	3,516*	62	−16
N Zealand	937	82	1,856†	78	−4
Norway	1,363	83	4,520	84	+1
Poland	258	96	910	70	−26
Portugal	614	65	2,120	71	+6
Spain	815	79	2,458	71	−8
Sweden	1,492	90	3,202	82	−8
Switzerland	1,782	68	4,311	60	−8
Turkey	171	61	591**	71	+10
UK	968	84	2,670	87	+3
US	2,738	40	6,714	46	+6

Notes: * 2004. † 2003. ** 2005. $PPP is a form of currency conversion making spends across countries more easily comparable.

Source: Organisation for Economic Co-operation and Development (OECD) Health Data 2008.

Latin, *quid pro quo* means 'something for something' or some sort of exchange of goods or services. This fits the language of economics nicely, whereby obtaining something that is worthwhile involves some sort of sacrifice, or a price to pay, even if that price is not determined in the marketplace. In fact, health care is riddled with quid pro quos, all of which we need to recognise if we want to save our publicly funded systems. Some quid pro quos we can do little about, the main one being that public financing of health care does not get rid of scarcity of resources, so choices have to be made. But others we can control. Even if we are convinced of the need for public financing, there remain various and large questions about how we can best organise health care. Despite political promises about 'protecting front-line services', we need to be clear about what this means. It could mean spending the same amount, but with a greater proportion of funds coming through private payments. It could also mean maintaining the budget, which would not keep pace with things like demographic change – so even promises to maintain spending means that cuts are coming. Either way, we need to gloss over what the politicians are saying and get more 'savvy' about rationing health care, ensuring that such care goes where it can do most good. This will lead to the ultimate quid pro quo; limits on health care resource availability mean that we have to put a value on our own and other people's health.

Scarcity and value

All societies limit what they spend on health care. Some spend more than others, but, at some level, such limits imply a value on life or health. More and more, we see controversial rationing decisions played out in the popular press. Should we be providing drugs for people with mild dementia? What about extending life for people with terminal cancer? What is such life extension for a mother would allow her to attend her daughter's wedding? The forthcoming credit crunch in health care, which will arise as governments roll back spending on public services, will only increase the frequency with which such questions are asked.

Underlying all of this is the notion of scarcity in the sense that we do not have enough resources to meet all of society's needs. Scarcity has always been with us, but, in the good times, we are not so focused on recognising this. But better management of scarcity is required to maximise lives saved and health gained. Scarcity simply means that there is an inevitability of choice, whereby in choosing to use resources to meet one need, we give up the opportunity to use those resources to meet some other need. The inevitability of choice, therefore, means that we are forced, as a society, to place value on health care, which also means we are either implicitly or explicitly placing values on life and health in different contexts.

For most other commodities, these notions of value are played out in the marketplace. Take food, for example. It could be argued that access to food is a more fundamental human right than access to health care. Yet no country has a National Food Service in the way that many have a National Health Service (NHS). Beyond setting some standards for food producers and supplementing the income of the less well-off, the delivery of food to individual members of society is largely left to the market. Yet, if food is so fundamental a commodity, why cannot the same be said of health care? The answer is that there are basic and persistent characteristics of the commodity we call 'health care' that make it susceptible to 'market failure', and thus more efficiently financed through the public purse, than just about any other 'good'.

The aims of this book, therefore, are to examine the notion of 'value' in health care, and, through discussion of how maximum value is best achieved, reveal to the reader how the value of their own health can be established, either from the perspective of government agencies making decisions about us or from surveys of the public in which the reader could theoretically be a participant. In managing resource scarcity, values are placed on the health of the public and what we want to achieve is maximum value. However, with most advanced economies having rejected the market as a route for the financing of their health care systems, we first need to explain why this rejection of the market has happened and whether it can continue to be justified in economic terms. But it does not end there, because scarcity still exists. Thus we need to examine the consequences that follow from the intervention of governments. In particular, we can review the evidence, showing how governments try, and often fail, to get best value for patients and the population from our publicly funded systems. Given this, what might be the ways forward and what do these mean in terms of what we as taxpayers and the governments that represent us say our health is worth?

From scarcity to value in health care

But how is this to be done? To start us off, in Chapter Two, you will be asked to suspend belief and think of health care as a 'commodity'. This will be strange to many people, but is not so far-fetched. It is a fact of life that, in the absence of any government intervention in health care, the societal response would be for a market to develop. In refuting those who continually come up with arguments to deregulate health care, therefore, our first task is to address the question of why the optimum value of health care is better *not* pursued within such a market framework. This is done in Chapter Two by comparing health care with food in justifying why public financing for health care is so crucial *for efficiency purposes*. Unfortunately, this does not solve the scarcity problem. We still have to decide as a society who gets what in health care, and, occasionally, who shall live and who shall die. Many clinicians and managers will be aware of this issue. Whether in public or private systems, we can only spend £1 or $1 once, and, effectively, a clinical decision is a purchasing decision. The rest of the book then reviews the main mechanisms put in place by governments to establish best value from these decisions, and thus how we can maximise equitable health and minimise deaths and morbidity from such decisions. In Chapters Three and Four, we address the issues around trying to reinstate some element of market forces within largely publicly funded health care systems. This is achieved mainly through some form of private (or out-of-pocket) payment by patients (which, its proponents often argue, will prevent frivolous use of the health care system) and through the promotion of 'internal markets' to at least try to impose some form of market-based discipline on NHS-type systems. The potential for more explicit rationing, through what economists would call economic evaluation, is then assessed in Chapters Five and Six, by outlining in general terms how we need to get to grips with the management of scarcity and then by describing, more formally, the main methods of 'economic evaluation' that exist. A major challenge for economic evaluation, and a crucial question we build up to, is how to place a monetary value on health. Recent attempts at doing this will be outlined in Chapter Seven and, thus,

—
5

some tentative 'answers' provided to the question 'What is your health worth?' The 'where now?' questions are addressed in Chapter Eight.

This is not a conventional textbook. I have tried to write it in a popular and accessible style for anyone who wishes to understand better, and from an economist's perspective, the reasons why we have the health care systems we have. Readers in Europe and countries such as Canada and Australia need to understand that simply having a publicly funded system is nowhere near the end of the story. There is a quid pro quo for this because public funding does not eradicate scarcity of resources and the need to make choices. As stated above, there are still huge questions to address in how we manage scarcity. People will still have to be excluded or to wait, but just not on the basis of ability to pay a market price or private insurance premium. If we get the clinical or policy choices right, we can minimise the suffering arising from exclusions and waiting lists, but we need to adopt the thinking and tools of economics to help us get there.

American readers need to make an even greater leap of faith. They need to understand why government intervention in health care is necessary from an economic efficiency perspective and that compelling all members of the public to participate in the same system through some form of taxation is an unfortunate, but minor, consequence of this. Without this recognition, all attempts at health care reform aimed at achieving the twin goals of affordability and universal access are doomed to failure. Therefore, in making these cases, it is important to warn the more serious academic reader that not everything I say is referenced. Where I attribute a statement or piece of evidence to a renowned health economics or health policy colleague by name, I have provided a reference to that piece of work in the further reading list at the end of the relevant chapter. I have also provided references to my own work, as detailed citations backing up the statements I make are available in these pieces. I hope the reader can live with this.

TWO

Market failure and health care

Introduction

In the UK, the National Health Service (NHS) has survived beyond its 60th birthday. Should we celebrate? Of course, there are lots of reasons as to why there is an NHS in the UK, as well as Medicare systems in Canada and Australia and similar such schemes in other advanced economies (with the exception of the US). However, this chapter focuses on the economic, as opposed to the moral or political, arguments. Although they stem from the discipline of economics, these arguments are just that – arguments. Nevertheless, while they may be contentious to some, it is fair to say that most health economists would subscribe to them.

Health care as a 'commodity'

As explained in the introductory chapter, to take our line of reasoning forward, it is necessary to suspend belief and think of health care as a 'commodity'. A commodity is essentially an item that can be exchanged in the marketplace; in other words, it is something for which there is both a demand and a supply, each of which will interact to determine the optimal amount produced.[1] Although this notion is anathema to many, it is vital to the case for significant government intervention in the health care 'market', allowing us to strip humanitarian and political arguments from the debate. To illustrate, one could argue that it is more of a fundamental human right to have access to food than health care. But why do we not have a National Food Service? Governments intervene in the food market to maintain production standards, providing income supplements where necessary. Such intervention is nowhere near as pervasive as in health care; the rest is left to the market. Make no mistake, if governments could do this for health care, they would.

The fact is that government intervention in health care is a global phenomenon – borrowing data from the table in Chapter One, see the selected examples of proportions of health care spending coming from the public purse in Table 2.1. The story we have to articulate is why this is the case. It is the nature of the commodity we call 'health care' that provides the explanation.

More particularly, health economists make the case for extensive government intervention on the basis of 'market failure'. Markets are merely an efficient way of transferring information (on prices as well as quantities and quality of goods) from producers to consumers. Technically, markets fail when they are so restricted in the function of transmitting information between consumers and providers that government intervention (for example, an NHS) becomes more efficient and more equitable. This is different from the more populist use of the term 'market failure', which refers to outcomes or consequences of market transactions that people dislike. We will focus on the more technical definition, as that is more important in explaining government intervention, health care being a classic case of information transmission breaking down in several ways.

The case for market failure in health care is not new. Specific aspects have been well rehearsed by Nobel laureates, such as Kenneth Arrow

Table 2.1: Total health expenditure in $PPP, and percentage of total that is public, for 1990 and 2006

Country	1990		2006	
	Per capita total expenditure on health	% of spend from public purse	Per capita total expenditure on health	% of spend from public purse
Australia	1,318	67	3,141	68
Canada	1,678	75	3,678	70
France	1,520	78	3,449	80
Germany	1,602	76	3,371	77
UK	968	84	2,670	87
US	2,738	40	6,714	46

Note: $PPP is a form of currency conversion making spends across countries more easily comparable.

in 1963, as well as many other social policy commentators. For more detailed arguments and all of the relevant references, see Donaldson and Gerard (2005). The problem, of course, is that these aspects tend to be forgotten. No doubt, as pressure on the public purse grows over the next few years, the arguments will be forgotten again as some policy commentators attempt to promote the case for deregulation of health care as a good thing. As the great Canadian health economist, Robert Evans, said about health care in 1997:

> ... advocates of private markets tend to make their arguments as if the last forty years has never occurred. The issues that were contentious in the 1950s and 60s are being dragged out again, with all sorts of old a priori arguments dusted off, repainted and presented as new thinking about the role of the private sector. (Donaldson and Gerard, 2005, p 31)

'Market failure' in health care: the tale of the duck-billed platypus

Aspects of market failure exist for many commodities. However, in health care, there are three sources of market failure, more than for any other commodity in society. When these are described below, the reader may naturally think of commodities that also possess a particular attribute. However, the key is that health care possesses all of them, and that is what makes it different. In the market-versus-non-market debates of the 1960s, Alan Williams, the eminent (now deceased, as of 2005) health economist from the University of York entered into a correspondence with an equally eminent economist, Dennis Lees (also deceased, as of 2008) from the University of Nottingham. In concluding his arguments about why government intervention in health care is necessary, Williams drew the analogy of the duck-billed platypus to illustrate how unique something can be in totality, even though some of its attributes, when looked at in isolation, are not:

–

9

It has a duck-type bill, a furry body like a mole, it lays eggs and it suckles its young. Now the argument you employ would run as follows.... Many birds have duck-type bills, and lots of animals have furry bodies, and as for laying eggs, this is common in birds and reptiles, and all mammals suckle their young, therefore the duck-billed platypus 'would appear to have to have no characteristics which differentiate it sharply from other ...' etc. I hope my point is clear. (Donaldson and Gerard, 2005, pp 31-2)

So, the point is that health care is distinct in the comprehensiveness of market failure associated with it, such failure arising from three main sources, each of which is described below.

The failure of health insurance

Without government intervention, an insurance market would develop to deal with unpredictable health care needs. Indeed, there are examples of such markets in various contexts around the world. However, insurance is particularly problematic in health care. First, fixed costs of billing and advertising tend to inflate premiums. Take the US, where one in four dollars of health expenditure is spent on administration. This prices some people out of the market who would otherwise have been willing to be insured at more actuarially fair prices (that is, premiums that reflect risk and not the add-on costs of administration). A larger, non-competitive company could spread such add-on costs across more enrolees, but equally such a monopolistic situation would present the opportunity for that company to exploit consumers. The only way to mitigate this problem without exploiting consumers is for government to intervene.

The second source of market failure in insurance is 'moral hazard', whereby the very act of becoming insured changes the way people behave. Because the concept of being insured encourages people to think that a third party (that is, the insurer) will pay, the market fails to input cost considerations into the decisions of consumers and providers, leading to cost inflation without much return in health benefits. This is the root of the continuing challenge of cost inflation in US health care, where entities that are one step further removed than insurance companies from the transaction (in other words, employers) pay many of the premiums; a combination of 'fourth-as-well-as-third-party pays' leads to spiralling resource use.

The problem exists in public systems, too, but government funding and supply-side controls (through the ability to limit human and capital resource) allow the lid to be kept on costs. A naïve observer would say that user charges could control costs. However, charges choke off demand only among poorer (and less healthy) people, are indiscriminate in the type of demand choked off (for needed as well as unneeded care) and do not control total costs anyway (as the system simply switches its care-giving powers to those willing and able to pay). It may also seem ironic that the greatest problems with cost control exist in those systems with the greatest prevalence of user charges, such as France and the US. This conundrum, along with other aspects of user charges, will be examined in more depth in the following chapter.

The 'caring' externality

In theory, well-functioning insurance markets target low premiums to those at low risk and higher premiums to those at higher risk. In health, those at higher risk tend to be less well-off, and thus unable to afford cover. Here, the market is working too well, and it does present a social problem because we tend to care about lack of access to health care among less well-off people. This is known as the 'caring externality'. It counts as market failure because societies struggle voluntarily to transfer contributions from those willing to pay to enhance others' access. Though not voluntary, taxation is a more effective way of achieving these transfers, achieving the double benefit of transferring income from rich and healthy to poor and unhealthy, as health tends to be associated with wealth.

Returning to the example of the food market, a caring externality exists there too. However, food does not possess the other two forms of market failure (listed above and below); hence the less pervasive forms of intervention. It could also be argued that societies could deal with caring through 'safety nets', such as the Medicare and the Medicaid systems for vulnerable groups in the US. However, in the US, this still leaves around one in six people uninsured or under-insured, which seems to go against the caring externality argument, and leaves the US as the main outlier among the advanced economies of the world in not being able (some would even say not willing) to ensure 100% coverage of its population in terms of access to health care. It will be interesting to observe the extent to which the Obama reforms to US health care can rectify this situation.

Consumer ignorance

Markets work well when consumers are well informed, which tends not to be the case in health care. Consumers are then protected in terms of quality through granting license to practise only to those with the qualifications to do so. By doing this, however, we indirectly give market power to professions. This requires what Evans has referred to as the 'countervailing power' of government, to promote a counterbalance to the market power of health professions in negotiating with these professions over rates of pay and provision of care.

What type of system?

The arguments above present a strong, many would say compelling, case for significant government intervention in health care, but does not prescribe exactly what form such intervention should take. Thus, although most advanced economies of the world seem to have adopted publicly funded systems, the details of these systems vary greatly. Generally, however, three main types of public funding exist, as shown in the box opposite.

Despite the differences between the systems, it is the similarities that are more significant for our purposes. Through different routes, there is an attempt at universal coverage of the population in all the schemes. This is generally achieved through some element of compulsion, where everyone has to pay taxes, or, in a Bismarckian-

Box 2.1: Main types of publicly funded health care systems

System	General description of source of funds and objectives
Beveridge	• Established in UK after Second World War, arising from Beveridge Report first published in 1943; forms the basis for current UK and other systems. • Funded from central or regional taxation. • Aimed at covering all inhabitants from outset. • If taxes are progressive, whereby higher earners pay a higher percentage of extra income earned to government, this system can be highly redistributive (that is, transferring resources from rich to poor).
Bismarck	• Often termed 'social insurance' and established in Germany in late 19th century (under Chancellor Bismarck); although much developed since then, it is still the basis for the current system in Germany (and other countries). • Funded from contributions from employees/employers, but now with state subsidies. • Initially aimed at providing a level of cover for payers. • Culturally, does not have same explicit redistributive agenda as Beveridge-type systems, although older people and unemployed are covered by other sources of funding, such as state subsidies.
Semashko	• Established in Eastern Europe under communism (and named after Nikolai Semashko, People's Commissar of Public Health in the Soviet Union from 1918 to 1930). • Funded from taxation, but now abolished and has developed to mirror Beveridge-type systems. • Given its origins, there is more emphasis within such a system on trying to achieve equality of services offered, although this is an issue in all systems, to a degree.

type system, where everyone has to contribute to a sickness fund. People seem to accept this compulsion to contribute, although a quid pro quo is that richer people in most developed countries are free to 'top up' their public coverage with private insurance and the UK allows physicians to supplement their public sector incomes by spending limited amounts of time practising in the private market.

The only advanced economy that does not allow top-ups is Canada, where it is illegal to pay privately for procedures that are covered via the public system. Canada is very proud of its one-tiered system, although it is important to point out that this applies only to (largely) physician and hospital services, which take up about 70% of health care spending. For the remaining 30% of health services, various types of private funding exist. This leads to multiple levels of coverage, inevitably meaning that poorer people end up with worse (and often no) cover for such services. Any claims about a superior Canadian health care system should therefore be taken with a pinch of salt.

Probably the final noteworthy characteristic is that 'insurance' in these funding systems is based on groups and not individuals, as in a classic private insurance model. This means that attempts are made to work out entitlements for everyone, and this inevitably creates tensions, as there are only limited resources available. A different kind of 'contract' is created between patient and payer in public as opposed to private systems. Generally, people have to wait longer in publicly funded systems because bed occupancy rates tend to be higher; peak flows of demand on the system are harder to accommodate when, on average throughout the year, 90% of beds are occupied. In the US, only about two thirds of beds are occupied on average; this is because, when patients are paying for private treatment, the 'contract' requires instant access to care once a diagnosis is made. Thus more 'spare capacity' is required of a private system to ensure peak flows of demand can be met. Another key aspect associated with publicly funded health care, however, ensures that standards are maintained in such a constrained environment. This is the characteristic of compulsion mentioned at the end of Chapter One, whereby, with the vocal middle classes locked in, any demands they place on the system in terms of quality maintenance end up being of wider benefit to more vulnerable groups in society. My view is that these groups would get left behind in terms of standards of service offered if the middle classes were able to opt out completely.

The lesson of compulsion is one that needs to be grasped by the US. America, of course, embodies a 'fourth way' of dealing with market failure not listed in Box 2.1; that is, it attempts to plug the gaps for vulnerable groups via Veterans Administration, Medicare for older people (and some other groups) and Medicaid (for those below a certain level of income). The rest is left to the market. This is a gross simplification of what is a very sophisticated health care system. For example, not everything is free at the point of delivery in the three public systems mentioned. The key point, however, is that around 50 million Americans fall between the cracks by being under-insured or having no private or public coverage. Fears abound as to what might have to be given up by those already covered if the US were to move to what is generally called a 'single payer' system so as to include those currently excluded. To 'sell' reforms to society at large, governments (not just in the US) tend to make them voluntary. The problem is, however, that voluntary reforms rarely work. All that happens with voluntary reforms in market-based systems is that those patients who are already low cost, and who would be likely to benefit from the reform financially, make the required change. Those who would not benefit financially stay in the more-established part of the system. Costs continue to rise, as will be seen in Chapters Three and Four.

Cultural and historical factors mean it is unlikely that any given country would move from one to another of the general systems described above. However, the basic point in terms of the content of this book is that all such systems, including that in the US, are faced with the same fundamental problem: once prices at the point of consumption of health care are covered (or heavily subsidised) by the state, claims on resources will be greater than the total resource available. Scarcity needs to be managed, leading to a set of common policy questions across such systems. Can user charges still be employed to moderate such claims and pressures on the system? Even though the arguments point strongly towards market failure in health care, can market forces still be used within a publicly funded system? As they are operated within a framework of public funding, such markets are known as 'internal markets'. If there are limitations to charges and internal markets, what then? What would be the economic approach to rationing care and thus facing up to the issue of establishing 'value' in health care? These questions are addressed in the remaining chapters.

Some final thoughts – and a toast

The arguments above rule out the market as the basis for a whole health care system, but do not rule out the use of market forces within an NHS-type framework. Recent governments have indeed shown this to be the case. The problem, however, is that governments, including the current UK government, are good on the rhetoric of evidence but not on the reality. What is the evidence that the extra billions the UK has put into its NHS in recent years have improved health? Have waiting targets improved health? Has greater private sector involvement improved health? Why have variations in health care provision continued, despite decades of evidence about their existence? Societies need to get much smarter in this regard. Later chapters, particularly Chapter Four, will sum up my views on the evidence.

Societies also need to wake up to recognising the scarcity of NHS resources and managing this scarcity. The economic approaches to such management are outlined in Chapters Five to Seven. The NHS used to be good at managing scarcity, but, with more and more money flowing into the system in recent years, our managers and medical personnel seem to have become less skilled in this regard. This may be good news for health economists like me, as a whole new generation requires educating in the subject. But on a more serious note, it is not a good situation for the NHS to be in; it represents a bad deal for the public and is the greatest threat to the sustainability of publicly funded health care over the next 60 years.

I would not claim, therefore, that the NHS is perfect. So, the toast I would propose is 'two cheers for the NHS at 60' and for all other publicly funded health care systems of the world. If we do what is proposed in the remainder of this book, we may be able to raise that to a full 'three cheers'. However, if we do deregulate health care, the market failures discussed above will come into play. Do we want to go down that route? Personally, I would propose no toasts to any non–NHS (or social insurance) system of health care financing.

Note

1 There are other aspects associated with goods being commodities, the most important of which is that the good concerned is not qualitatively different no matter who produces or provides it; gold is gold, orange juice is orange juice, and so on.

Further reading

Arrow, K.J. (1963) 'Uncertainty and the welfare economics of medical care', *American Economic Review*, vol LIII, no 5, pp 941-67.

Donaldson, C. and Gerard, K. with Mitton, C., Jan, S. and Wiseman, V. (2005) *Economics of Healthcare Financing: The Visible Hand* (2nd edn), London: Palgrave Macmillan, chs 2 and 3.

Evans, R.G. (1984) *Strained Mercy: The Economics of Canadian Medical Care*, Toronto: Butterworths, chs 1-4.

Evans, R.G. (1997) 'Going for the gold: the redistributive agenda behind market-based healthcare reform', *Journal of Health Politics, Policy and Law*, vol 22, pp 427-65.

THREE

Charging the public: exception or anomaly?

Introduction

One of the first questions a reader might ask at the end of Chapter Two is, "Given these apparently quite sensible arguments about market failure in health care, why then do many governments still operate a system of charging people for care at the point of use?" This would indeed appear, on the face of it, to be an apparent contradiction to the points made in Chapter Two. However, such user charges are often inherited or are nominal, having been introduced by governments as a political mechanism to make it look as though those who are using (and often portrayed as 'abusing') the system are being made to pay for it out of their own pockets as well as being subsidised by the wonderful taxpayer. Therefore, as examples, charges tend to be levied on items such as prescription drugs and visits to family doctors. Of course, it is never those wonderful taxpayers, to whom governments are trying to appeal, who are portrayed as abusing the system; it is always some other person. It is important to lay out the arguments against user charges so as to dismiss this as a way forward in getting maximum value from health care.

Every country has a different way of implementing user charges, but, as has been pointed out, a common feature is that they really do represent a minor source of revenue for health care funding (less than 10% in most countries), despite the attention they attract. The real question, then, is why *not* user charges? More precisely, what are the arguments against their more widespread use? Regular fiscal pressures in most countries lead to frequent debates about extending the implementation of user charges, and the health care credit crunch will be no exception. However, user charges will not

---

save our publicly funded systems, and indeed will act to undermine them. There is much evidence to support this argument, and there is virtually unanimous agreement about it among the experts. Yet, politicians, and the occasional clinician, keep coming up with user charges as a suggested cure for health care ills. I am not sure we can stop this, but the arguments contained in this chapter might help.

The popularity of user charges

Under severe fiscal strain, it is natural for politicians to opt for 'solutions' that appear to make intuitive sense; that by imposing a charge on health care use, such use will be moderated and pressure on the system relieved. User charges in different guises are often seen as innovatory in this regard. However, the real innovation is in the myriad of terms that politicians employ when describing what are essentially 'user charges'. Popular ones, emanating from the field of insurance, are 'co-payments' and 'cost sharing'; another one is 'diversifying the revenue stream'. But they are all different forms of user charge.

On the face of it, it seems very powerful to say, "Why not let people spend their hard-earned money in whatever way they like? Surely this relieves the public system of a burden rather than placing one on it?" Neither of these is true, unfortunately. User charges are an idea that is intellectually dead, but keeps coming back to threaten our publicly funded health care systems, and have thus been classed by leading health economists in Canada as a policy zombie. Occasionally, the zombie has to be slain, so the remainder of this chapter contains my brief attempt at doing so.

The fallacy of composition

Social scientists would say that proposals for user charges in health care suffer from the fallacy of composition; that is, the assumption that what happens at the level of the individual will happen at the level of the whole system, in this case the health care system. There is no doubt (and studies have shown this) that some users will respond to charges by reducing demands on the health care system. Indeed, one of the largest studies in health economics, the Rand Health Insurance Experiment, led by Joe Newhouse (Harvard) and Willard Manning (Chicago), provides very strong evidence to support this. But costs will not be saved. Why not? Because physicians, faced with reduced demand by one group and with a target income in mind, will simply provide more services to those who present. Combine that with the fact that those who choose not to present are likely to be poorer and more in need of care, and we end up with a system incurring the same costs and meeting less need than before.

One only has to look to the US to see this. The US makes the most widespread use of user charges in its health care system, and yet it faces the most difficulties in controlling health care costs of any country in the world. France provides the best example of this in Europe. Studies in the US and Canada have shown that when demand on the system is reduced, it is indeed poorer people whose demands decrease. And, because the poor are more likely to be ill, they suffer. Demand for needed care is reduced just as much as demand for unneeded care, which has been shown in ambulatory care for children and in the use of essential drugs among older people. So, the user charge is a blunt instrument. Not only that, if reduced demand for needed care develops into a more serious problem later on, that episode will end up costing the system more in the long run.

Furthermore, in any one year only a small percentage of the population accounts for the majority of health care costs. For example, in 2002, the US Agency for Healthcare Research and Quality estimated that 49% of health care costs were incurred by only 5% of the population and 64% of health care costs were incurred by only 10% of the population. This is because people in each of these groups are seriously ill and require high-cost procedures. It is doubtful that user charges would be levied for such procedures. They would have little effect anyway, as, at this stage of care, it is the physician who is calling the shots; that's what they are trained to do. But this also provides a major clue as to how to control health care costs.

Can we exempt people?

User charge proponents always say that some people can be declared eligible for exemption from user charges, thereby reducing unfairness. But how do we decide who is eligible for exemption and why create a whole new (and costly) bureaucracy for this? Also, with those who are exempt from user fees being able to access care as before and those who are not exempt also being able to access care because they can afford the charge, how is this going to reduce pressure on the system? There is no doubt that there are some things currently available in health care that patients should be asked to provide for themselves. For example, hospitals are not hotels, and some optional, non-health-related services could be scaled back, charged for or brought by patients themselves.

What are we trying to achieve?

Most countries adopt strong equity objectives for their health care systems, usually along the lines of trying to achieve equal access for equal need. In trying to achieve such a policy objective, user charges would be disastrous. As has been seen, they would not reduce demand overall, but would compromise the equity objectives of our health care systems. For any form of financing health care, there is always an alternative, and, in the case of user charges, the alternative would usually be some form of taxation as a source of funds. In countries with progressive taxation systems, rich people pay a greater rate of taxation on extra income earned, thereby subsidising the care of poorer groups, especially as poorer people are more likely to need care anyway. Thus, given the association between income and health, all that user charges do is make poorer people pay more than they would under a system funded from progressive taxation. This is effectively a transfer of income from the poor and sick to the rich and healthy.

Proponents of user charges may argue that there is simply not enough in the taxation pot to continue to support our health care systems in the ways that we have before. However, these systems have endured severe funding crises in the past. Furthermore, as a mere economist, I can only point out the consequences of different funding regimes. Despite my personal opinions, as an economist, I am comfortable with individuals having the right to spend their own money on health care. But this should come with two conditions. First, proponents of such policies should come clean and admit that their proposals involve changing the resource allocation process within publicly funded systems towards one based, at least in part, on willingness and ability to pay. Second, politicians who support the introduction of any such scheme should seek societal approval for it at the ballot box.

Medical savings accounts: another way of placing decision burden on the 'consumer'

The medical savings account (MSA) is a recent innovation that has received much press attention. But while MSAs seem intuitively to have much potential, they are, unfortunately, riven with challenges. Under such schemes, each person/family would have an amount deposited in their account (in the UK, by government) at the beginning of the year. They can spend this on minor health care items (like visits to the GP), although (problem number one) the boundaries for this have yet to be defined. If the money in the account runs out, individuals pay for such minor items in full from their own pocket up to a maximum amount. If the account does not run out and there is money left at the end of year, it can be carried over, used to pay for long-term care insurance or even pocketed, depending on the scheme. The expensive treatments, in hospitals, would still be provided by the state as now. The idea, once again, is to make consumers more aware of health care costs. How can there be any downsides? Well, apart from the issues of defining what such money can be spent on and the administrative costs of setting up millions of such accounts, there are others related to our theme of equity.

First, consumers/patients are not very good judges of when and when not to go to the doctor. Studies of user charges in the US and, more recently, in Quebec, have shown that people respond to paying at point of use by reducing their demands for essential as well as less essential care. This has knock-on effects on emergency room use, which means costs are not saved. As with user charges, putting the decision-making burden on the consumer may not be a good idea.

Second, MSAs are likely to be regressive. Countries that have used MSAs have found that poorer people and older citizens have problems keeping within the limits of their accounts. Better-off, and generally more healthy, folk tend to have money left over. Effectively, and again as with user charges, what is observed is a redistribution of income from poor to rich. Poor people do not use health care when they should, while rich people get to use their surplus on something financially beneficial to them.

These problems might be overcome if adequate adjustments could be made to the amount in people's MSAs according to their age, sex, presence of chronic diseases, socioeconomic status and so on. But, as noted above, countries with experience of such accounts do not seem to have been able to do this. Furthermore, if all these adjustments were made to make the system 'fair', one might question the point of doing so. Not much changes, except that the consumer now has more (apparent) financial control, which, as already pointed out, may not be a good idea.

Top health policy analysts from Canada, Evelyn Forget, Raisa Deber, and Leslie Roos (2002), have conducted excellent research to assess the costs of MSAs in a publicly funded health care system. They have shown that, due to the concentration of health care costs, a small number of people each year are high-cost patients whose care costs are covered, while most people do not consume much care at all (so effectively governments would be giving them money that would either cost society more or have to be taken out of the health care system). Hardly anyone would be in the 'corridor' in between, where the MSA is activated, and, incidentally, where reliance is also placed on people being well-informed 'consumers'.

To date, MSAs have not taken off. Ultimately, they are voluntary. In this situation, only those likely to gain financially (that is, infrequent users of health care) will opt in, while those unlikely to gain would stay in the mainstream of the system. Overall, therefore, simple economic logic would dictate that such schemes would have little effect on the costs of the system overall. One exception is the area of management of chronic disease, where one would expect some patients to have accumulated a significant degree of knowledge about their condition. Should savings accounts go further than this group of people? I would say not. Perhaps they should not even go that far, as many people with chronic diseases will also be old and frail and carry multiple pathologies; perhaps being too vulnerable to act in the role of 'the good consumer'. But watch this space.

An exception to the exception: lower-income countries

One of the great ironies of health care financing is that, despite the strong equity-based arguments against user charges, they are highly prevalent in low-income countries around the world. However, this is not a conspiracy against poorer people but more a reflection of circumstance. As economies develop and eventually begin to consider funding more coherent health care systems, the main challenge will be in having the state infrastructure in place to collect funds. Many lower-income countries lack the kind of formal economy that is recognisable in many higher-income countries, which makes collection of funds (in the form of taxes) difficult. Such countries, therefore, tend to start by taxing groups that are easy to capture, such as civil servants and other public sector employees, with the remainder of the population facing either severely limited health care access or paying privately.

This is illustrated, at least in part, by Figure 3.1, which I have adapted from the excellent work of Normand and Busse (2000). As economies, and subsequently infrastructure, develop, the aim of most health care policy makers becomes that of moving from the right-hand to the left-hand side of the figure where more and more payments are made into a collective fund that may be private but is more often public. This is all well and good, but what are the masses of least-well-off in the world to do in the meantime? Over the past 20-30 years, microfinancing has grown to provide basic packages of health services that can be funded by poor people paying small sums to a collective, sometimes with subsidies and often run as a social business (that is, where surpluses are reinvested into services), mimicking what we in the West might think of as the role

Figure 3.1: Types of financing and their implications for user charges

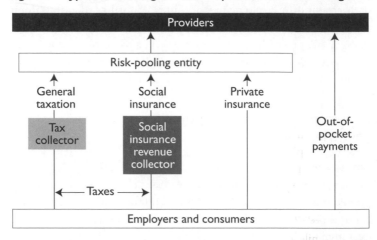

of government. From the recent work of people such as Dowla and Barua, we now know that the poorest people will pay into such institutions. Whether this is a case of markets adapting or reparation of a form of market failure is not clear, but it would certainly seem to be the case that microfinancing has, in part filled a gap that governments and large financial institutions either would or could not.

Conclusion

If societies want to control health care costs and at the same time reduce the moral dilemmas that budget-busting drugs pose for society, the most important thing to recognise is that most decisions in health care are taken by providers, even in the US. Again, we are back to the notion that a clinical decision is a purchasing decision. Governments have to take courage and target the supply side of this complex market. It is wrong, unfair and ineffective to try to limit consumer and patient access through user fees, and also to dress it up as something that enhances access. Nevertheless, the 'realpolitik' of lower-income countries means that a substantial proportion of funding in the early development of a health care system will come from such payments. That aside, as systems become more advanced, alternative and effective ways to involve clients and the public more generally in health system decision making and in making good choices about health and health care need to be found. If we want to limit access to supply-led services, it needs to be acknowledged that many of the actual choices in health are made by the health care professionals who manage and provide care. As patients, we would as a matter of course want such professionals to be doing their utmost for us on a one-to-one basis. However, the question remains as to whether, at the broader levels of general patterns of practice and provision of programmes of care, professions and institutions (such as hospitals) can be influenced via health care reform and economic appraisal to better meet societal needs for health care. Is the general (or family) practitioner, as family doctor and friend, best placed to balance the care budget rather than focusing on individual 'consumers'? These are the issues to be discussed next.

Meanwhile, by way of a summary on user charges, if societies want a financing mechanism consistent with what they want to achieve in health care, there is another way: taxation. No doubt the user-charge zombie will be back. When it returns, and if you are asked to comment on it, you may wish to refer to the arguments above. For now, let us move on to other potential ways of reforming health care.

Further reading

Donaldson, C. and Gerard, K. with Mitton, C., Jan, S. and Wiseman, V. (2005) *Economics of Healthcare Financing: The Visible Hand* (2nd edn), London: Palgrave Macmillan, ch 6.

Dowla, A. and Barua, D. (2006) *The Poor Always Pay Back: The Grameen II Story*. Bloomfield CT: Kumarian Press Inc.

Evans, R.G., Barer, M.L., Stoddart, G.L. and Bhatia, V. (1993) 'Who are the zombie masters, and what do they want?', Vancouver: Centre for Health Services and Policy Research, University of British Columbia.

Forget, E.L., Deber, R. and Roos, L.L. (2002) 'Medical savings accounts: will they reduce costs?', *Canadian Medical Association Journal*, vol 167, pp 143-7.

Manning, W.G., Newhouse, J.P., Duan, N., Keeler, E.B., Leibowitz, A. and Marquis, M.S. (1987) 'Health insurance and the demand for medical care: evidence from a randomized experiment', *American Economic Review*, vol 77, pp 251-77.

Newhouse, J.P., Manning, W.G., Morris, C., Orr, L., Duan, N. et al (1981) 'Some interim results from a controlled trial of cost-sharing in health insurance', *New England Journal of Medicine*, vol 305, pp 1501-7.

Normand, C. and Busse, R. (2000) 'Social health insurance financing', in E. Mossialos, A. Dixon and J. Figueras (eds) *Funding Healthcare: Options for Europe*, Buckingham: Open University Press, pp 59-79.

Tamblyn, R., Laprise, R., Hanley, J.A., Abrahamowicz, M., Scott, S., Mayo, N., Hurley, J., Grad, R., Latimer, E., Perrault, R., McLeod, P., Huang, A., Larochelle, P. and Mallet, L. (2001) 'Adverse effects associated with prescription drug cost-sharing among poor and elderly persons', *Journal of the American Medical Association*, vol 285, pp 2328-9.

FOUR

Reform, privatisation and those damn doctors

Introduction

To many, the very notion of a market in health care is anathema, or, at the very least, a 'contradiction'. A more measured approach might be to question the place of markets in our publicly funded systems. Thus, rather than being a contradiction in terms, the phrase 'markets and health care' becomes a conundrum, to be informed by theory and evidence.

Part of that conundrum has been examined already. In Chapter Two it was argued that the market is not a good basis for an efficient, never mind equitable, system of health care financing. Moreover, in Chapter Three, we saw that, equally, user charges are neither equitable nor efficient. These arguments notwithstanding, the discussion in this chapter moves us on to recognising that market failure does not preclude competition on the supply side of health care – for example, among different providers, such as hospitals, competing for public funds. These are so-called 'internal markets', whereby people's care is still tax-funded, but entities within the system, such as hospitals, have to compete for patients and, thus, for these funds. Proponents of such internal markets would say that they retain some of the theoretical advantages of full-blown markets while mitigating many of the problems outlined in Chapters Two and Three. Indeed, this recognition has informed the reform of many health care systems around the world during the past 20 years. Unfortunately, these reforms have not been informed in turn by robust evidence. We review the evidence here such as it is and consider why so many systems are obsessed with emulating the US experience, in this case its attempts to inject managed care into the health care market.

Public finance or public provision?

Public financing of health care relates to how the funds are raised, whether through insurance premiums, taxes and so on. Provision varies, and is more about the institutions through which care is delivered. So far, the arguments in previous chapters have been about justifying public financing of health care, not about public provision. This is why the apparent contradiction becomes more of a conundrum – there may be scope for markets, or competition, on the provision side, which then requires evidence to establish the degree to which this should occur.

Figure 4.1 illustrates a matrix of cells that represent the combinations of health care financing and provision that can occur. With the exception of user charges, the health care systems in most advanced economies are largely publicly financed with no competition in terms of that dimension – as depicted by cells 1 and 3. The renowned UK health economist, Tony Culyer (1991), has referred to this as 'demand-side socialism'.

However, as the figure illustrates, this does not rule out the possibility of competition on the supply side, that is, among providers such as hospitals. Indeed, this is the policy direction (moving from cell 1 to 3) that many governments have recently adopted in so-called attempts at enhancing the efficiency of their health care systems. Such policies have become known as 'internal markets', retaining 'demand-side socialism' but introducing 'supply-side competition'.

Figure 4.1: Competitive/non-competitive mix in health care financing and provision

		Financing	
		Non-competitive	Competitive
Provision	Non-competitive	(1)	(2)
	Competitive	(3)	(4)

Given that this has happened, the crucial question then becomes, 'What does the evidence say about internal markets?'

Evidence on internal markets

Health authorities as purchasers

Internal markets were initially adopted in countries such as the UK, New Zealand and Sweden, but versions of them now exist in several other countries. Briefly, money allocated from central government went into the hands of health authorities (HAs), as in the previously existing systems in these countries. The difference was, however, that, under internal markets, providers had to compete to win contracts from HAs. Through competition among providers, the aim was to improve quality and reduce costs, not only of medical care but also other services provided through hospitals. Less quantifiable objectives were for HAs to avoid getting bogged down in micro-management and to realign the balance of power away from large provider units (that is, hospitals) towards purchasers with a more population-oriented perspective.

In the UK, there seems to be little doubt that opportunities for competition did exist if one looks at the number of providers within a 30-mile radius of an HA. For example, in one major region of England (the West Midlands), only 8% of acute hospitals had a monopoly of their main surgical specialties within such a radius. Generally, however, other factors counteracted the opportunities for competition; for example, directives from 'the centre', crude contracting mechanisms (which meant that large amounts of money were simply handed over as in the old system), the enormity of the task and a general risk aversion among purchasers with respect to not wanting to destabilise a local provider by reallocating finance to some other provider.

In Sweden, with health care organised mainly at the level of county councils, there were fewer central directives and more scope for change. It was also easier to evaluate the impact of the changes as some counties took up internal markets while others did not. The evidence, here, shows that cost savings of up to 13%, along with productivity enhancements, were achieved in councils with internal markets relative to those without.

Returning to the UK reforms, one should not be too pessimistic about the impact of the internal market. The well-known health policy commentator, Professor Chris Ham, has described what happened to health care in London in 1991. Given the population and number of hospitals, particularly relatively expensive teaching hospitals, in London, this is precisely the place where one would have expected the UK reforms to have an impact. Indeed, this is what happened. Almost immediately after the reforms were introduced, purchasers located on the outskirts of London stopped sending patients to central London hospitals, referring them instead to local hospitals in less costly and more accessible surrounding areas. These resource movements were sufficient to create problems with respect to the sustainability of some central London hospitals and led to the suspension of the internal market in London and a review of health services in the UK capital, led by Sir Bernard Tomlinson. The review gave greater priority to community and primary care services, while London's hospitals were given more resources to enable them to cope with the changes. Eventually, hospitals were closed or rationalised. It could be argued that such rationalisation led to little real change, while others may say that a combination of market signals and government management led to a more orderly process of change than would otherwise have been the case. Yet the internal market still had an impact. It is claimed that other major cities experienced similar changes, but at a slower pace than in London.

General practitioners as purchasers

Unique to the UK was an additional proposal that general practices of a certain minimum size, if they so wished, be given more responsibility for the purchase of hospital services. They were given a budget to purchase elective inpatient services, outpatient services and diagnostic tests on behalf of their patients, similar to health maintenance organisations (HMOs) in the US. Later, some practices evolved into 'community' or 'total' fundholders, extending the range of services that were purchased by the fundholder. The aim was that general practitioners (GPs) would also choose care for patients on the basis of both cost and quality. Patients remained free to change practice, budget allocations being suitably adjusted. Where general practices opted for budgets, HAs had their budgets reduced by the amount allocated to these general practices for 'buying in' hospital services.

The voluntary nature of this scheme made it difficult to evaluate. However, evidence of the impact on referrals to hospitals is reasonably encouraging – reduced waiting times in England and reduced referral numbers in Scotland for some groups.

Carol Propper and colleagues (1998) have shown, through rigorous regression analyses, that market forces, measured by variables such as numbers of NHS providers in a given area and market share accounted for by a provider, have had an impact in reducing prices charged to fundholders across eight common procedures. It appears that fundholding practices provide more services (such as outreach clinics run by hospital clinicians) after they became fundholders. However, whether this shift in activity from secondary to primary care is attributable to fundholding per se is, again, not entirely clear.

Other considerations relate to the high administrative costs of fundholding, due to diseconomies from having such costs present in several small units as opposed to spread across a larger HA. Because of this, the UK's Audit Commission raised the question of whether fundholding was worthwhile. Analysis of equity impacts showed that the pattern of use of GP and inpatient services remained stable over the period 1990/91 (before the UK reforms) to 1993/94 (three years after). Use was still slightly in favour of the poor, after adjusting for indicators of need. Thus, equity (or inequity) in health care delivery remained largely unaffected by health care purchasing.

UK developments under New Labour

In 1997, in England, the New Labour government replaced HA and fundholding purchasing with primary care groups (now trusts), which are responsible for purchasing most hospital, community and primary care for their populations. These primary care trusts (PCTs) cover all practices, and cooperation rather than competition was encouraged between purchasers and providers. PCTs are typically much smaller

—

than HA purchasers but are still run by professional managers, which means that GPs are no longer involved in direct purchasing. Encouraging cooperation does, to some extent, dilute the incentive effects on PCTs to manage resources in the ways GP fundholders did, especially when combined with central government initiatives, such as national service frameworks and national treatment guidelines, to which trusts are expected to adhere. Although difficult to interpret in terms of attribution to these reforms, increases in hospital activity were not as great as during the period 1989/90 to 1996/97, with the total number of GP consultations falling between 1996/97 and 1998/99. A more sophisticated, but still limited, case-weighted activity index, measuring units of resources used per unit of activity, showed improvements in 'efficiency' during the period of the internal market and has fallen since. Numbers of people on waiting lists for treatment did, however, decline, from 1.16 million in 1997 to 1.039 million in 2001. Whether this is due to greater cooperation, increased funding, or some other reason is not clear. For example, some have suggested that shorter waiting lists resulted merely because, among the plethora of performance criteria introduced since the 'abolition' of the UK internal market post-1997, those relating to waiting times are more easily measured.

Despite the apparent success of shorter waiting lists, Julian Le Grand (2002) (a former government health adviser) has attributed the lack of success in other areas at least in part to a lack of the incentives that would result from competitive pressures. It could be argued, then, that the purchasing function has been made weaker, with consequent (possible and slight) adverse effects. The recent (re?)introduction of Foundation Hospitals in the UK, may, in part, be a response to this problem. Such hospitals are ranked according to how well they perform and, if ranked in the lowest category, they are given a period of time to reach certain targets. If they fail to meet these targets, private management teams and those from other (say, neighbouring) hospitals can compete to take over the management of the 'failing' hospitals. Those in the top category are given more freedom to raise capital and, therefore, further develop services. This 'franchise' scheme remains unevaluated. Where it seems to differ from the earlier version of the UK internal market, however, is that more emphasis has been put on providers rather than purchasers, thus weakening the purchasing function even further. The extent to which (now smaller) purchasing units will be able to exert their authority against (still) large 'three-star' Foundation Hospitals remains unclear. It could be characterised as leading to less of a focus on population health, as more resources are 'sucked' into acute services that may or may not be efficient. The incentives for acute hospitals to suck in such resources are greater than ever. This is due to a financing scheme called 'payment by results', which means that a fixed payment is received for each case admitted. This amount differs by the type of case (a hip replacement is more expensive than a hernia repair, for example), but each payment is based on the average cost of treating any such case. Given that the extra costs of admitting more patients will not amount to this full average cost, hospitals could be making considerable surpluses from admitting more and more patients. This is further reinforced by many hospitals having funded major capital developments via private finance initiatives (PFIs). These PFIs can be paid for only by having more people, and thus more money, in hospitals. More than ever, those arguing for population and public health perspectives are up against it – at least in the UK.

Does the 'for-profit versus not-for-profit' literature help?

In the absence of data on the cost-effectiveness of public funders such as HAs purchasing services from private hospitals, there is more of a focus on for-profit versus not-for-profit hospital literature. A recent paper from Canada, by Gillian Currie and colleagues, explored the relevance of the literature on for-profit versus not-for-profit hospital care to publicly funded systems. The key to this study was that, rather than select articles and reports to help make the case for one side or the other in this controversial debate, the authors sought to systematically review the literature in order to provide a balanced view of the evidence. Thirty-four studies were identified and most of these found no difference between for-profit and not-for-profit full-service hospitals with respect to relative costs, quality of care or efficiency, a conclusion that is contrary to the more selective reviews that focus on the results from either favourable or unfavourable studies, depending on whether or not they are promoting for-profit provision.

Why should the relevance of such literature to health care in Canada, or elsewhere for that matter, be considered? First, it should be pointed out that the literature concerns full-service hospitals and this is different from the type of involvement of private providers that is being considered in the context of most publicly funded systems. To illustrate, some of the studies referred to above have shown for-profit US hospitals to be more costly than not-for-profit hospitals, other things being equal. However, the US context is different. The main objective of for-profit hospitals, of course, is to make a profit. This is partly achieved by selling services, the characteristics of which are not necessarily fully accounted for in empirical studies. In a market-orientated environment, such hospitals cannot be criticised for selling a service for which consumers are willing to pay. This is like criticising Rolls Royce or BMW as being inefficient because they sell expensive cars. The fact that many for-profit hospitals show higher margins of surplus than not-for-profit hospitals would seem to indicate that they are, in some sense, more efficient, even if more costly.

In many countries, the legislation allows for public bodies (HAs) to purchase care from private providers. The effect of this may be quite different to the experience of for-profit versus not-for-profit hospitals in the US, but, as mentioned above, there are no studies about cost-effectiveness in this particular context. Dogma rules while there is a lack of rigorous research to help the public decide what is right and what is wrong.

Lessons from America?

The main health care reform innovation in the US over the past 20 years has been that of managed care, essentially in the form of HMOs and preferred provider organisations (PPOs). In short, the aim was for these developments to induce more cost-consciousness in the US population and in health care providers, with consumers paying something towards the costs of care and HMOs/PPOs paying for costs of any referrals (so having to pay for comprehensive cover).

HMOs and PPOs may also have had a limited set of providers to whom patients could go, with patients having to pay more if they wished to visit any other provider.

There are many studies of managed care and it is difficult to generalise because of the myriad of arrangements for HMOs and PPOs in the US, but the main message is that managed care has led to lower costs and utilisation, albeit with some two-way selection going on, with lower costs arising either because low-cost people (i.e. people with fewer health care needs) select such plans or the plans select them. More competitive areas seem to have done better at reducing prices as a result of greater HMO penetration.

At the system level, the shortcomings of managed care are reflected in evidence that, over the years, no major reform of the US system, including managed care, has abated cost increases. Health care premiums in the US rose by 11% in 2001 and by 13% in 2002.

It seems, then, that, in such a system, consumers are free to choose whatever plan best suits them. This means that those who want lower-cost care, perhaps with more emphasis on prevention, will choose HMO-type plans, while those who want higher-cost care, and maybe those in poorer health, will enrol (or continue to enrol) in fee-for-service (FFS)-type plans. Indeed, other analyses have shown that the market is responding to such a situation with increasing enrolment in more traditional Blue Cross and Blue Shield plans since the mid-1990s and, to compete with this, managed care plans are now offering less restrictive and higher-cost packages. This may be a good thing, but does counter any evidence that HMOs reduce, or even stabilise, costs overall.

On the supply side, hospital mergers, partly to combat managed care, have led to higher prices being charged back to insurers and consumers. The evidence for managed care never was that strong. But now, with the combination of demand and supply-side effects and the related, and growing, concern for quality, it seems that the managed care revolution is no longer being sustained. Instead, a counter-revolution has occurred, comprising the dreaded alliance of providers and consumers, and managed care appears to be dying out.

President Obama, beware. Once again, the key to reform in the US is compulsion, locking people into a single universal system.

Constitutionally, this may be impossible in the US. With people free to choose, which to a great degree they still are under recent Obama legislation, they will continue to choose in ways that benefit them financially. If so, the costs of the US system will continue to rise. In this respect, the US has much more to learn from Europe (and Canada) than the other way round.

Paying doctors

One way in which financial incentives have been shown to work is in influencing the behaviour of individuals as opposed to institutions like hospitals. The most studied area has been that of financial remuneration of physicians. This is a key area because it is physicians who make most of the resource-committing decisions in health care. If different forms of remuneration influence these decisions, we have a powerful tool for achieving efficiency and value in our health care systems.

An excellent example of this is provided by the Copenhagen case study described in Box 4.1. Originally, primary care doctors in the city of Copenhagen were paid on a capitation basis, which means that, for each person registered with that primary care doctor, the doctor will receive a fixed annual pre-payment. In this case study, the payment system was changed in order to introduce some elements of FFS. FFS is more of a piece-rate form of payment, where physicians are remunerated 'per consultation' or surgeons 'per operation'. FFS is often criticised as being a bad form of remuneration because it encourages overprovision of services. This has been shown, for example, in cases of surgical services, with rates of common operations being higher in systems that reward surgeons via FFS than those in which surgeons are paid monthly in the form of a salary. However, there may be cases where we actually do want doctors to provide a lot of some services, a good example being vaccinations for young children. In Copenhagen, FFS was used to encourage primary care physicians to provide services that otherwise would have been carried out in the more expensive hospital environment. The results in Table 4.1 show that, for the most part, it worked. The rates of service provision are indexed to 100 so that changes can easily be

Box 4.1: Paying doctors: Copenhagen case study

The method of remunerating GPs in the city of Copenhagen was changed in October 1987. Previously, payment had been by capitation (that is, the GP would receive a fixed payment per annum for each person registered with their practice). The system changed to one of part capitation and part fee for service (FFS). Fees were introduced for general items, like face-to-face contacts, and also for specific items, such as:

- 40 special services (for example, cervical smears);

- 40 special laboratory services to be performed in the practice (for example, estimation of haemoglobin concentration);

- some preventive services (for example, immunisations).

A before-and-after study was carried out to examine the effects of introducing these changes. The remuneration of GPs in Copenhagen county, where the new system was already in place, was used as the control.

expressed as percentages. They show little change in Copenhagen county, but do show significant changes in Copenhagen city where the remuneration change took place. The first line in Table 4.1 shows that rates of face-to-face consultations did not change much. This is to be expected, as the decision about whether to attend a consultation is largely taken by the patient. There were more changes where decisions about services are more likely to be taken by the physician, with more services being provided in primary care settings and fewer by specialists or in hospitals.

Some health economists would interpret these results as evidence of supplier-induced demand. Supplier-induced demand is thought to arise from asymmetries in knowledge between suppliers (in this case, doctors) and consumers (in this case, patients), which may give doctors the power to over-recommend services for which they are remunerated. Despite the unadulterated glee that economists often

Table 4.1: Estimated changes in number of contacts and specific activities per 1,000 enlisted patients in March and November 1988 compared with that in March 1987 in Copenhagen City and change in Copenhagen County by type of contact

Type of contact	Copenhagen city			Copenhagen county	
	March 1987	March 1988	November 1988	March 1988	November 1988
Face-to-face consultations	100	112.7	104.4	105.5	104.9
Diagnostic services	100	138.1	159.5	105.3	107.6
Curative services	100	194.6	194.8	106.0	115.0
Referrals to specialist	100	90.1	77.0	99.4	98.1
Referrals to hospital	100	87.4	68.4	97.1	102.1

Note: All changes were statistically significant.

Source: Krasnik et al (1990)

express when detecting supplier-induced demand, there is actually not a lot of evidence of its existence. A less negative interpretation might be preferred – that medical doctors are human after all. They respond to incentives just like the rest of us. General practitioners may know that prevention of cervical cancer saves costs and that the service is likely better provide by them, but they require incentives to act on this thinking. Also, such results could be interpreted as a result of simple market economics, whereby if an adequate price for a good is offered, supply of that good (in this case diagnostic and curative services) will be forthcoming.

The key here is to decide on objectives and then keep a range of remuneration options open to ensure that the objectives are met. Broadly, it is not wise to remunerate hospital physicians by FFS, and in this respect some major countries, such as the US and Canada, are very wrong. Others, like the UK, where hospital doctors receive a salary (along with other bonus-type rewards as their careers advance) have it broadly right. In primary care it is good to maintain blended systems, with FFS for some activities and capitation for others. Sometimes, target payments can work too. It is also useful to keep the option of paying quite high salaries in primary care to encourage doctors to practise in locations to which it is difficult to recruit, or, indeed, further upward adjustment of budgets paid to practitioners in such localities.

Conclusion

In summary, market failure refers to the challenges markets face in transmitting information between producers and consumers in ways that lead to optimal resource allocation. As the data show, most high-income countries seem to have taken on board, either explicitly or implicitly, the market failure arguments as applied to health care. However, it may not be as contradictory as it seems to introduce market forces on the provider side of the health care market. Indeed, many countries have done so, and some such experiences, largely those of the UK, have been considered here. It may sound contradictory in itself to imply that there are some good things about competition and then to criticise the failure of US policy on managed care.

But, it is important to be clear about this. Context is everything, the context into which market forces are introduced being crucial to the discussion. First, a regulated system of the purchaser–provider type does seem to have had a positive impact: philosophically, someone is more likely to be looking after the population's interests, but the potential may not have been realised, partly because such reforms were not in place long enough and because efficiency is not the only objective (hence the small impact). In the UK, GP fundholding probably had the greatest impact, but was seen by New Labour as the epitome of the internal market, and was thus abolished in 1997. From a UK perspective, the danger is of seemingly moving to a more provider-dominated system than ever, with a weakened purchasing function. This continues to serve the acute–medicine model, which is outdated because our population is healthier than ever before. This means we need to get away from the view that we are fit one minute, then seriously ill the next, miraculously treated, and thus returned to full health. The kinds of condition we are more likely to be dealing with are frailty in old age, learning disabilities, mental health, alcohol and drug dependence, chronic disease, dementia and the like. But the incentive systems and resulting care plans are just not geared up for this, serving neither efficiency nor equity and perpetuating our failings in public health.

Despite this critique, politicians will continually claim success for the reforms they have introduced such as reducing waiting times, providing more choice for patients or linking GPs' pay to quality of care provided. But despite the lack of an evidence base for such policies in the first place – for example, we still have no information on how long patients would be prepared to wait for treatment given that the resources devoted to waiting time reductions could have other health-enhancing uses – a key point is that a major part of the context is that, almost invariably, such reforms are accompanied by large spending increases. The point made by Maynard and Bloor in their incisive article about the UK health reforms of the early-to-mid-1990s still stands today:

> The reforms were introduced with a considerable increase in NHS funding. Disentangling the short-term effects of the funding and the medium-term effect of managerial reform from the NHS reforms themselves is impossible. The market reforms in the UK are not an end in themselves, but a potential means of improving efficiency while cost control is maintained. It is necessary to distinguish between, on the one hand, the political need to claim success and, on the other hand, evidence of improved efficiency – which is incomplete at best, and ambiguous and uncertain at worst…. The mere 'redisorganization' of the service's structures which has preoccupied politicians for decades, does little to ensure that resources are allocated efficiently in a cash-limited NHS that provides universal coverage. (Maynard and Bloor, 1996)

Some may hold on to claims in favour of market-based reforms and waiting time targets by quoting evidence that England has preformed better than Scotland in productivity measures since adopting (or retaining) such initiatives. However, as David Hunter (2008) has so eloquently argued in his recent book, such comparisons say nothing about relative quality of care across the two countries; widespread 'gaming' of such targets has been acknowledged and policy makers have simply directed different priorities towards their health care systems in Scotland and England.

Second, and again this may sound contradictory, but in the system, where one might expect competition to work best (i.e. that of the US), it seems to have failed. Problems of risk selection and the fact that consumers have freely opted out of managed care into higher cost plans have led to a continuation of rising costs. This is the essence of the problem – that these very basics of competition (freedom and tailoring of packages to risk) act against competition ever achieving the desired goal (of maintaining quality and keeping costs down). Ironically, a restricted type of competition, where consumers are locked into the broader system and cannot opt in and out, may work better.

A challenge for all systems is to ensure that physician behaviour is harnessed so as to best serve the notions of value and efficiency for patients and the population. Clinicians are best placed, especially if they are budget holders, to deliver the care plans that best meet the needs of patients and serve the system efficiency, and we know they can be financially induced to do this.

The key is to establish objectives. It is then likely to take a mixed system of financial incentives to meet these objectives. Some countries have more work to do on this than others. The challenge for public systems is to strengthen the purchasing function so as to allow the purchasers (who could be family doctors) to move resources around the system more in line with population need. Although such doctors tend to operate in smaller units than health authorities or primary care trusts, there is nothing to stop them acting in consortia. In addition, their medical professional status may permit them to challenge more readily the power of the acute sector. The message for the US system remains as always; strengthening purchasing will not do much in a system where missions impossible seem to be:

- to agree on objectives for the system;
- act accordingly in terms of broader health care system reform; and

- accept that some amount of sacrifice (most likely by better-off members of society and also by health care providers) may be required to achieve such reform.

Further reading

Culyer, A.J. (1991) 'The normative economics of healthcare finance and provision', in A. McGuire, P. Fenn and K. Mayhew (eds) *Providing Healthcare: The Economics of Alternative Systems of Finance and Delivery*, Oxford: Oxford University Press.

Currie, G., Donaldson, C. and Lu, M. (2003) 'What does Canada profit from the for-profit debate?', *Canadian Public Policy*, vol 29, pp 227-51.

Donaldson, C. and Gerard, K. with Jan, S., Mitton, C. and Wiseman, V. (2005) *Economics of Healthcare Financing: The Visible Hand* (2nd edn), London: Palgrave Macmillan, chs 7 and 8.

Ham, C. (1996) *Public, Private or Community: What Next for the NHS?*, London: Demos.

Hunter, D. (2008) *The Health Debate*, Bristol: The Policy Press.

Krasnik, A., Groenewegen, P.P., Pedersen, P.A., von Scholten, P., Mooney, G., Gottschau, A., Flierman, H.A. and Damsgaard, M.T. (1990) 'Changing remuneration systems: effects on activity in general practice', *British Medical Journal*, vol 300, pp 1698-701.

Le Grand, J. (2002) 'Further tales from the British National Health Service', *Health Affairs*, vol 21, pp 116-28.

Maynard, A. (2005) *The Public-Private Mix for Health*, Abingdon: Nuffield Trust/Radcliffe Press.

Maynard, A. and Bloor, K. (1996) 'Introducing a market to the United Kingdom National Health Service', *New England Journal of Medicine*, vol 334, pp 604-8.

Propper, C., Wilson, D. and Soderlund, N. (1998) 'The effects of regulation and competition in the NHS internal market: the case of general practice fundholder prices', *Journal of Health Economics*, vol 17, pp 645-73.

FIVE

The fiscal future of health care: an economist's rant

Introduction

This is the most embarrassing chapter of the book, for two reasons: it involves me ranting in a rather negative manner; and, then, what I propose as a potential way forward is in fact really quite mundane, despite its impeccable logic. My starting point is that, as a consequence of market failure, the allocation of health care funds according to geographically defined populations, and usually adjusted for measures of need, is now the norm in the most advanced economies of the world – the basic notion of which is a fixed funding envelope that can never meet all possible claims made on it. You will recall that scarcity in the health care context refers to not having enough resources to meet all needs; the situation described above is therefore an example of scarcity. The fundamental challenge of managing scarce health care resources for maximum population health still exists, but seems to be consistently denied by the actions of those who govern and administer our health care systems. Hence my rant begins, with the logic as follows. First, let us rule out user charges and related tools for rationing care that place financial and decision burdens on patients. Second, although sensible structures and incentives are needed, all the fiddling about with these aspects over the past 20 years has not really got us very far. Hello! In a cash-limited system, as is the case for health care in most advanced economies, whatever entities are put in place as a result of health care reform, they all have to manage scarcity.

The problem is that governments have not responded well to scarcity. Indeed, it could be argued that the reforms discussed in Chapter Four represent a form of scarcity denial. In response to health care 'crises', it is easier to keep reorganising the system rather than face up to the hard choices that need to be made once scarcity is recognised. The result is that health care systems frequently end up in financial crisis, followed by severe and arbitrary cutbacks to clinical care that go too far in the opposite direction and lead to embarrassing surpluses; 'boom and bust' abounds.

This argument is developed in the following section. At risk of repeating some of the material from Chapters Three and Four, this section outlines other common 'innovations' in health that give the appearance of managing scarcity, but in fact represent even more scarcity denial. In the interests of positivity, the chapter goes on to outline a framework for managing scarcity, around which commissioning and planning of health services could be based. This framework is remarkably simple and brimming with common sense – indeed, readers may expect health service managers and clinicians already to be applying such a framework to their decision-making processes on a daily basis. But readers should also be wary of economists who claim their proposals are based on common sense; consequently, this chapter will consider why health organisations have problems implementing such frameworks.

The 'scarcity denial' rant: when in doubt ...

Whenever governments get around to addressing challenges to their health care systems, they historically employ three main strategies, as follows.

... reform

Reform almost sounds like something that is desirable in and of itself, something that can only ever be an improvement over the status quo and should never be questioned. However, many countries have grappled unsuccessfully with the types of reform outlined in Chapter Four, the UK being no exception. Broadly, Scotland and Wales have gone from having more integrated health boards and authorities to internal markets and back again. Indeed, they are now thinking of integrating health and social care budgets at the local level. New Zealand has done the same thing. England has tried different forms

—

of commissioning since the original internal market model and is now introducing combined primary care trust (PCT) executives (reminiscent of the old-style health authorities) and practice-based commissioning (rather like fundholding, but without the purse strings attached, which, as intimated in Chapter Four, may be worse than before). In the province of Alberta in Canada, the notion of geographically defined health authorities emerged just over 10 years ago, but has now been reversed, with the role of commissioner being taken on by a provincial-level body. This is happening just as Canada's largest province, Ontario, is moving towards a health authority-type system.

Thus, many societies stumble from one non-evidence-based reform to another, and end up going round in circles, albeit with the best of intentions. A common factor among these reforms is the creation of entities that have to manage scarce resources. Yet, in over 60 years of the National Health Service in the UK, such entities have never been issued with comprehensive guidance or tools to do this that extend beyond political rhetoric and management speak.

... keep spending

There is no question that overspending in publicly funded health care systems is the norm. But how does it happen? The simplest answer, of course, is that health professionals and organisations simply respond to incentives put in front of them. More often than not, governments bail out overspending health organisations. The incentive is, thus, to overspend, but not by too much. Such overspends, as a percentage of turnover, are often not that large, so, some may say, the problem is not that serious.

Although there is some logic to this argument, there is a degree of denial here; after all, are we not concerned about *how* the money is spent?

The answer to this question is surely a resounding 'yes'. If governments are not concerned about this, why do they continually attempt to reform the system? Many governments would argue that this has something to do with maintaining financial balance while providing high-quality, safe and effective services, despite the fact that most economies do not seem to be able to implement a set of incentives that prevent the inexorable march of patients into the most expensive part of the system – the black hole of the acute care sector. In Canada, for example, there is a disconnection between primary and secondary care, the incentive being to 'refer on' from the former to the latter. In the UK, there are powerful incentives to get people into hospitals, with strong providers and weak purchasers combined with heavily centralised policy and a reliance on non-evidence-based targets aimed at things like waiting lists. With little or no knowledge about how long patients are willing to wait, and despite competing demand for resources in other areas, many countries continue to throw more and more money at these 'initiatives', pushing even more cash into the hospital sector. However, these days could be over. As with our economies in general, the dream of continuous growth in health care is seemingly just that – a dream. Now is time for payback.

... and/or create a national health technology assessment agency

Some countries have sought to address the problem of scarcity in their health care systems by creating health technology assessment (HTA) agencies. Perhaps the best example of this is the National Institute for Health and Clinical Excellence (NICE) in England. From an economic perspective, the remit of these agencies is to assess interventions for 'cost-effectiveness' and reduce geographic inequalities in health care provision. However, national guidance on the provision of new therapies will, according to a ratio of *incremental* costs to incremental health gain relative to current provision, result in increased rather than reduced costs. In England, where such guidance is compulsory, resources to fund the implementation of NICE guidance must be found (by PCTs as budget-holders, not by NICE) from elsewhere because costs are incremental. Such guidance may not fit with the priorities of the PCTs themselves, given all the other demands on their budgets. National guidance does not, and indeed cannot, make holistic judgements about the range of services to be funded in any given locality. Furthermore, there may be a temptation among PCTs simply to add the cost consequences of NICE guidance to their expenditures. If so, the guidance will simply be inflationary, something that health economists such as Amiram Gafni and Steve Birch (1993) from McMaster University have warned about for several years now.

Please note that I am not using these arguments to condemn national HTA bodies. It is important to remember that such organisations are looking in detail at the evidence for certain interventions, preventing duplication of effort and challenging the system to respond to what appear to be sound, evidence-based assessments. Nevertheless, they deal only with a fraction of the NHS budget, and do not necessarily look at what PCTs want them to look at. It could be argued that in the UK the NHS spends £100 billion or so each year that is largely unscrutinised.

This gives a strong clue as to where to go now. Fundamentally, NICE 'guidance' needs to be managed, and sometimes challenged, locally. This has to be combined with resource management, clinical judgement and accountability at the local level that requires strong commissioning based on sound frameworks. NICE is now moving to aid commissioners in these respects, encouraged by high levels of UK government (see Box 5.1). Without giving this support, HTA agencies are only playing at dealing with scarcity.

Box 5.1: The disinvestment agenda

'NICE should be asked to issue guidance to the NHS on disinvestment, away from established interventions that are no longer appropriate or effective, or do not provide value for money' (Chief Medical Officer Annual Report, 2005).

"NICE has an excellent track record in identifying and recommending the most effective new treatments. But we need to ensure that we balance this with better advice on unnecessary and ineffective interventions that can be stopped" (Andy Burnham, UK Health Minister, September 2006).

Where now?

The reality is that health economics needs to be developed at the local as well as the national level. However, at the local level, the analytical resources do not necessarily exist to conduct sophisticated analyses of the sort undertaken by HTA agencies and a wider range of factors may need to be considered at the local level than in a general national-level assessment of a drug or technology. Thus, if HTA agencies, like NICE, and academic health economists are to maximise population health from the resources available, a paradigm shift is required in order to fit the economics to local NHS entities rather than impose technically sophisticated, inappropriate analytical frameworks and the results gained from such frameworks. This point is eloquently argued by Ruth McDonald (2002) in her seminal work on the use of health economics in the NHS in England. Chapters Six and Seven elaborate on these more sophisticated frameworks, but for now the point is that the quid pro quo for local health organisations is that they would still have to be willing to work within a framework that recognises scarcity and thus the need to make choices.

It is possible to use certain guiding principles in conjunction with a pragmatic framework. Part of my argument, however, is that, although it is hard to argue with the impeccable economic logic of a set of principles and a framework, both of which are straightforward in themselves, they are not applied commonly and systematically in health care. In order to improve this situation, we need to ask why this is the case, and the resulting solutions require an element of pragmatism. Nevertheless, without recognition and management of scarcity, the sustainability of our publicly funded systems has to be called into question.

The principles: 'opportunity cost' and 'the margin'

An economic approach to priority setting simply has to adhere to two key economic concepts: 'opportunity cost' and 'the margin'. Opportunity cost refers to having to make choices within the constraint of limited resources; certain opportunities will be taken up while others must be forgone. The benefits associated with forgone opportunities are opportunity costs. Thus, we need to be familiar with the costs and benefits associated with various health care activities. Marginal analysis refers to the fact that cost and benefit assessment is best addressed 'at the margin', where the focus is on the benefit gained from the next unit of resources, or benefit lost from having one unit less. If the marginal benefit per pound spent from, say, an elective heart operation programme is greater than that for an elective hip replacement, resources should be taken from hips and given to hearts. But where does this allocation process stop? Do we wipe out the hips programme completely?

This is best answered by referring to the sequence of diagrams in Figure 5.1. Let us assume that we can measure both costs and benefits (that is, health gains) from treating hearts and hips in terms of money, as on the vertical axis (see Figure 5.1a). A further assumption is that these programmes and all others are operating at maximum 'technical efficiency' in the sense of there being no waste in the system. Minimisation of technical inefficiencies has been explored in the literature, and can be incorporated into the framework, but is set aside for now for purposes of illustration. First, we activate the economic (and reasonable) assumption of diminishing marginal

Figure 5.1: Marginal analysis

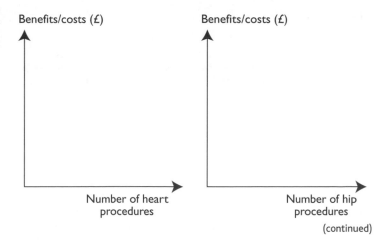

a. Benefits and costs can be measured in £s

Benefits/costs (£)   Benefits/costs (£)

Number of heart   Number of hip
procedures   procedures

(continued)

Figure 5.1 (continued)

b. Treat those who benefit most

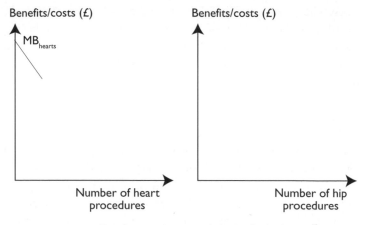

c. Continuous downward-sloping 'curve'

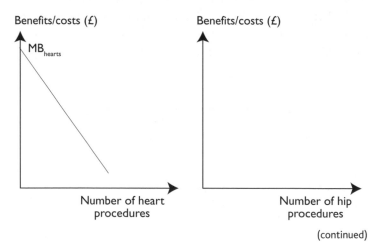

(continued)

benefit, whereby physicians and surgeons treat people in order of magnitude of benefit gained. Thus, those who gain most from a heart operation will be treated first (as in Figure 5.1b). Accordingly, if we increase the number of patients treated over a set period of time, we are adding patients who benefit less and less from the procedure, leading to the downward–sloping marginal benefit (MB) line for

Figure 5.1 (continued)

d. Same for hips, but different slope

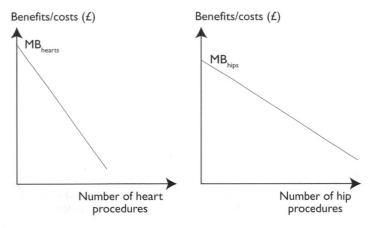

e. Equal marginal costs

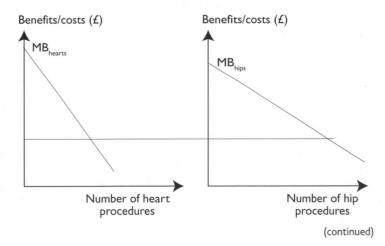

(continued)

hearts (Figures 5.1c) and a corresponding one for hips (although the hips line has a different slope, Figure 5.1d). If we also assume for purposes of illustration that the cost of each procedure is constant and equal for all patients receiving the procedure (Figure 5.1e), cutting back on hips from its starting point (Figure 5.1f) will increase its ratio of marginal benefit per pound spent, while expanding hearts

Figure 5.1 (continued)

f. Where do we go from here?

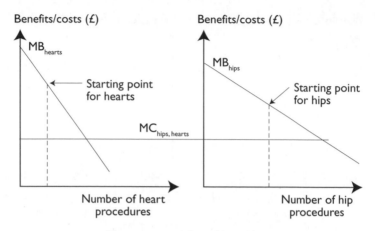

g. Move resources from hips to hearts,
until ratios are equal (as indicated by dotted horizontal line)

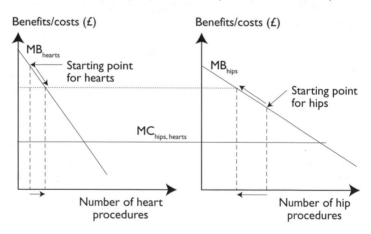

will diminish its equivalent ratio (that is, we will get an increasingly lower rate of return in terms of health gain for each additional pound invested in hearts). To maximise total patient benefit derived from the combined budgets of the two programmes, the process of reallocation should continue until the ratios of marginal benefit to marginal cost (MC) for the programmes are equal (Figure 5.1g).

Thus, we would never consider a total elimination of either service. The application of economics here concerns the balance of services, not the introduction or elimination of a service in totality. Examining changes at the margin is central to attempting to make the most of the resources available by deploying them either across or within programmes so that relevant outcomes are achieved in the best manner possible. Below, the issue of who would make such decisions is addressed, although the main point is that decisions are made no matter who makes them.

Operationalising opportunity cost: a pragmatic framework

A proposed framework, based on opportunity cost and marginal analysis, is outlined in Box 5.2, where the scenario of hearts versus hips has been used for effect. The framework provides a structured way of thinking about planning service delivery either at the level of a programme (such as diabetes) or services for a whole population (see the further reading list at the end of the chapter for examples of my own and others' experiences of using and developing such a framework).

The starting point is to examine how resources are currently spent before focusing on marginal benefits and marginal costs of changes in that spend. Known by the rather cumbersome term of programme budgeting and marginal analysis (PBMA), the framework can be used at the micro level (that is, within programmes of care), at the meso level (across services within the same general area of care) or at the macro level (across all services and programme areas within a single health organisation). At its core, the approach can be operationalised by asking five questions about resource use as listed in Box 5.2. A hugely important point to note is that the starting point is *resources*, not need (which would be the natural point of departure for many health care professionals). The satisfying result of this is that need met from available resources would be maximised. Indeed, the wider the range of services covered (for example, with health and social services under one budget), the better the result.

The first two questions in Box 5.2 pertain to programme budgeting, while the last three concern marginal analysis. The

Box 5.2: Programme budgeting and marginal analysis: the five questions

PBMA addresses priorities from the perspective of *resources*:

1. What *resources* are available in total?

2. How are these *resources* currently spent?

3. What are the main candidates for more *resources* and what would be their cost and effectiveness?

4. Are there any areas of care within the programme that could be provided as effectively but with fewer *resources*, thus releasing those resources to fund candidates from question 3?

5. Are there areas of care that, despite being effective, should have fewer *resources* because a proposal (or proposals) from question 3 is (are) more effective in terms of the *resources* spent?

underlying premise of programme budgeting is that we cannot know where we are going if we do not know where we are. If the health care budget is fixed, opportunity cost is accounted for by recognising that the items for service growth (question 3) can be funded only by taking resources from elsewhere (questions 4 and 5). Resources can be obtained from elsewhere by increasing technical efficiency (for example, by treating the same conditions differently and achieving the same health outcome at less cost, see question 4), or allocating resources more efficiently (for example, by treating entirely different conditions to achieve a greater health outcome at the same cost, see question 5). Technical efficiency can be achieved through various schemes commonly known as 'efficiency savings', such as 'lean thinking' and eliminating unwarranted variations in costs of procedures. Question 5 is more difficult because it involves taking resources from some groups of patients to give to others. However, the key is that all of this can be done 'at the margin' by considering the amounts of different services provided. Although in reality quantitative data on marginal benefits are often lacking in many areas of health care, it is the clear and logical *way of thinking* underpinning the PBMA framework that is of prime importance. The more technical ways of estimating costs and benefits are outlined in Chapters Six and Seven. However, these techniques can also be applied, although perhaps more crudely, in local health organisations that still have to manage scarcity.

Of course, readers may assume that governments add real resources incrementally to health organisation budgets year on year anyway, and that top priority service development is funded in this way. However, given that such increased funds are unlikely to cover all proposed growth areas, and that scarcity will continue, the principles of PBMA still apply. In effect, and at the other extreme, the whole base budget (£100 billion in the UK), as opposed to the annual increment, is available for reallocation. With the public services credit crunch coming, annual incremental increases are likely to level off anyway.

Managing scarcity by project management

This may be the least interesting part of the book, albeit one of the most necessary. Put simply, implementation of the framework described above relies on good principles of project management, as listed in Box 5.3. A practical toolkit by Mitton and Donaldson, listed in the further reading section at the end of this chapter, describes these stages in more detail. Another way of looking at Box 5.3 is in terms of the evaluation cycle assess–plan–implement–evaluate–assess and so on.

First, the nature and scope of the PBMA exercise needs to be defined; are we dealing with a disease grouping, an age grouping (like services for frail, older people) or something even wider than these (such as priority setting across disease areas)? Despite technical challenges, this way of thinking can be applied at any level of health care where resources are scarce, in other words, all of them – clinical, programme, practice, Trust, health authority and national. Second, the programme budget requires compilation. All this represents is a statement of how resources are currently spent in each relevant programme or parts of a programme. It can take many forms, and examples of national and local programme budgets can be seen below.

—

Box 5.3: Seven stages in a PBMA priority-setting exercise

PBMA stages	
1. Determine the aim and scope of the priority-setting exercise.	Assess ←
2. Compile a programme budget (that is, a map of current activity and expenditure).	
3. Form a marginal analysis advisory panel and stakeholder advisory groups.	

4. Determine locally relevant decision-making criteria:
  a. decision-maker input;
  b. stakeholder input (for example, service providers, patients, public).	

5. Advisory panel to identify options in terms of:
  a. areas for service growth;
  b. areas for resource release through producing same level of output (or outcomes) but with fewer resources;
  c. areas for resource release through scaling back or stopping some services.
	Plan

6. Advisory panel to make recommendations in terms of:
  a. funding growth areas with new resources;
  b. decisions to move resources from (5b) to (5a);
  c. trade-off decisions to move resources from (5c) to (5a) if relative value in (5c) is deemed greater than that in (5a).
	Implement

7. Validity checks with additional stakeholders and final decisions to inform budget-planning process.	Evaluate

A key issue, then, is to think about who is going to be making decisions or recommendations. With this kind of approach, careful consideration must be given to the make-up of the advisory panel, and to the various stakeholder groups whose views and advice will be sought. The balance is in obtaining representation while keeping the decision-making process manageable by not having to consult too large a group. While the specific composition of the advisory panel will be dependent on the question under consideration and the scope of the exercise, it is likely to comprise a mix of clinical personnel and managers, and may include patients or members of the public. Data and financial personnel are also key resources in the decision-making process. Too often health organisations work in silos, with clinicians set against management, finance functions merely serving to balance the books without communicating with public health and so on. History (the way things were done in the past) becomes the main driver behind the allocation of resources. PBMA is a great way of getting over this, bringing all these functions together to ask the most relevant question of all: 'How can we maximise benefit to the population with the limited resources available to us?'

In evaluating options for change, we need to make decisions about the criteria against which such options will be judged. Otherwise, it will be difficult to know how decisions were arrived at. Another advantage of using such criteria is that they can be applied to all the options competing for resources (naturally, there is no room here for golf-course deals); if the process is violated, the reason for this will be more obvious. As for the degree to which such criteria have been met, local knowledge can be supplemented with evidence from any number of sources. Thus, formal economic evaluations of the sort outlined in Chapter Six need assessment, and other sources of information, such as national and local policy documents and health care professional and public surveys, can be used to assess the impact of shifting resources. In the end, however, it is the members of the advisory panel who are charged with recommending whether resources should be shifted. Where evidence is lacking, group members are required to base recommendations on their own 'expert'

—

opinion, or on whatever such opinion can be obtained within the relevant timeframe.

This will not be an attractive option to those who prefer to base decisions only on the most rigorous evidence. However, scarcity of evidence does not eliminate scarcity of resources – decisions still have to be made; hence the importance of conducting a final round of consultation with a wider group of relevant stakeholders, in order to test the validity of the recommendations and increase the prospects of gaining acceptance for the suggested changes.

Challenges to managing scarcity

On a positive note, research on the use of PBMA to date has shown that managers and clinicians want to work with more systematic processes. Nevertheless, significant challenges remain. The bottom line is that if the organisation is not ready and does not possess the leadership required to implement such a framework, it will not work. Stuart Peacock and colleagues (2006) have spent several years researching the implementation of PBMA and have come up with a checklist to help organisations to meet the challenges (see Box 5.4). The checklist is drawn from a process of synthesising evidence and experiences of conducting or evaluating approximately 30 such studies in the UK, Australia and Canada, as well as experience of conducting over 70 priority-setting workshops with managers and doctors over the past 15 years since 1995.

Pragmatic considerations in priority-setting processes relate to establishing organisational objectives; understanding organisational context and ensuring organisational 'readiness'; establishing an appropriate priority-setting advisory panel; and, ensuring that the implementation of results is feasible. These form the basis for the checklist for pragmatic considerations in resource management and priority-setting processes shown in Box 5.4. The objectives of the organisation (health authority, commissioner, provider and so on) should be established at the outset of any priority-setting exercise. Establishing these objectives requires careful consideration of three interrelated issues. First, managers and doctors within the organisation may have multiple objectives (such as clinical effectiveness, equity, cultural appropriateness and so on). Second, objectives should reflect the local decision-making context, but also be compatible with policies at higher levels (hierarchical objectives). Third, organisations will have different short- and long-term objectives (inter-temporal objectives), and differences that may occur across all levels of decision making.

Perhaps the strongest challenge to any explicit, evidence-based, priority-setting process is that of organisational context and behaviour. An understanding of organisational culture and internal politics is necessary to implement such a process successfully. Strong management leadership and clinical champions are required to drive any priority-setting process; if leadership and champions are absent, it is unlikely that the process will be successful. Priority-setting studies should be undertaken in a context of *relative* organisational stability (considering that flux is the norm rather than the exception in health services), with some degree of coherence in long-term strategies for planning across health services. Institutional boundaries, such as budget and service delivery boundaries, should be clearly established. A key question is whether stated objectives are achievable within current institutional boundaries. If not, the objectives being considered should be revised in the short term. Incentive and sanction mechanisms, including remuneration and funding mechanisms, should be identified, and their potential impact on resource management decisions examined.

International experience has highlighted the central role of the 'advisory panel' in priority setting, whose function it is to make recommendations for reallocating resources within a given budget to better meet organisational or health system objectives. The importance of this has been discussed above. A further key point is that the advisory panel should receive training in the principles of priority setting, a necessary prerequisite if the stakeholders are to have ownership of the process. Community stakeholders can play an integral part in the process, including defining appropriate criteria for decision making based on community values and ensuring that the needs of specific groups within the community are addressed (for example, cultural appropriateness). However, some caution should be exercised with the use of stakeholder views as a proxy for community values because of the danger of tokenism and professionalisation.

The implementation of priority-setting results will only occur if a decision-making culture that considers costs, outcomes and trade-offs between alternative uses of scarce resources has been established. It may not be practically feasible to change some services in the short term, for example, in cases where services are jointly provided by more than one agency. These services may be potential candidates for change in the future, when the means to overcome institutional boundaries have been more fully explored. Successful application of priority-setting methods requires a degree of integration in funding and priority-setting mechanisms. If priority-setting mechanisms conflict with funding mechanisms at the local or regional level, or with budget-setting mechanisms within provider organisations, it is unlikely that priority-setting exercises (such as programme budgeting and marginal analysis) will lead to changes in the allocation of resources.

Crucially, managers and doctors must 'buy in' to the key concepts that underpin economic processes like PBMA. Tensions between doctors and managers and differences between medical and managerial cultures have existed since the earliest provision of organised health care; their historical roots are well documented. In a resource allocation context, doctors could be caricatured as taking the role of patient advocate while managers take the corporate, strategic view. Commentators from both sides of the cultural divide have identified an apparent paradox in this uneasy doctor–manager dynamic. On the one hand, efficient (and in the case of the NHS, equitable) health care delivery requires doctors to take responsibility for resources and to consider the needs of populations, not just individual patients. It also requires managers to focus on health outcomes and to become more patient-centred. On the other hand, modern health care (and the patient) may best be served when both professionals behave according to type, pitted one against the other in perpetual yet ultimately productive conflict, although I am not convinced about this. Indeed, a similar argument is used to justify market competition, where the best outcome arises when neither buyers nor sellers have overall control in the marketplace.

—

Box 5.4: Checklist for pragmatic considerations in priority-setting processes

1. Establish the organisational objectives:
   a. multiple objectives (effectiveness, equity, trade-offs between objectives);
   b. hierarchical objectives – micro level (provider), local, macro level (regional), national;
   c. inter-temporal objectives (short-term, long-term).

2. Ensure organisational 'readiness':
   a. leadership and ownership (managers, providers, consumers, community);
   b. timing and stability (organisational reforms);
   c. institutional boundaries (budgetary, service fragmentation/ integration);
   d. incentive and sanction mechanisms (financial, managerial).

3. Establish an appropriate advisory panel structure:
   a. advisory panel composition (service managers/providers, consumers/community);
   b. roles and responsibilities (values, decision-making criteria, evaluation of services);
   c. training of key stakeholders (information provision/ education);
   d. community participation and values (values, decision-making criteria, specific needs).

4. Ensure that implementation of results is feasible:
   a. desirability of resource reallocation (desire to reallocate resources, ownership);
   b. feasibility of resource reallocation (ability to reallocate resources, institutional boundaries);
   c. funding and priority-setting mechanisms (degree of integration/conflict).

PBMA offers a practical solution to this paradox. There is now an emerging consensus that a successful partnership between medicine and management is most likely to be achieved through joint leadership and the alignment of goals. To accomplish 'a convergence of cultures', the well-known health care management commentator, Chris Ham (2003), suggests it is necessary to 'harness the energies of clinicians and reformers in the quest for improvements in performance that benefit patients'. The PBMA process has the potential to do precisely this; it provides a practical framework that can facilitate the alignment of goals and joint working in several ways.

The methodology of PBMA both requires and values equally the contributions of doctors and managers. For example, different models of medical practice each play a legitimate part at different stages in the PBMA process. Although heavily dependent on physicians themselves, a reflective model of medical practice that draws on tacit knowledge borne of individual clinical experience is invaluable in formulating the criteria by which investment and disinvestment candidates will be assessed, in generating those candidates, and in subjectively assessing the benefits gained or lost from proposed marginal shifts in resource allocation. At the same time, doctors bring essential critical appraisal skills to bear on the evaluation of investment and disinvestment options, and the integration of clinical evidence from systematic reviews. Managers, on the other hand, in addition to providing the more obvious organisational, operational, financial and strategic management skills necessary for PBMA, can crucially ensure success at critical stages of the process through cooperation, negotiation, delegation, teamwork and persuasion, skills generally more highly developed among managers than doctors. Managers can also ensure that the local and national policy context exerts an appropriate level of influence on the final choice of priorities. This is no less important than the clinical evidence base if PBMA is to lead to real change in service delivery.

A major advantage of PBMA arises from its transparency and inclusivity. Contextual information, evidence and subjective judgement are explicitly presented, evaluated and recorded. This makes it far more difficult for any professional group to defend (or reject) a stance simply through obfuscation, unsubstantiated assertion

—

or the exploitation of ignorance. Implementation of an explicit evidence-driven process that directly incorporates the economic principles of opportunity cost and the margin is also likely to minimise legal intrusion into public policy making, in the sense that such a process is defensible. In addition, the perspectives of doctors and managers are both mediated and illuminated by a range of other viewpoints garnered from service users, the public, nursing and other professions allied to medicine, epidemiologists, and often professionals from other non-health agencies.

The most important and far-reaching benefits of PBMA for the doctor–manager relationship may come through a subtle form of interdisciplinary education. In ways that may not be immediately apparent, joint participation at each stage of a PBMA exercise can lead to a shared understanding of each other's cultures. The net result may be a shared appreciation of opportunity cost, of the need to focus on resources *and* health outcomes, and the need to balance clinical autonomy with financial responsibility. Sustainable publicly funded health care systems depend on a mature recognition of the need to manage scarcity. PBMA can help achieve this precisely because it bridges clinical and strategic decision making.

Do we have the data?

Where do we start with this? Having said that various UK NHS entities have survived for 60 years with limited guidance or support, a significant advance in recent years has been the development, by the Department of Health, of national-level programme budgeting data for England. These data can be used to examine spending by any PCT across 23 programme budgeting categories (mostly disease-based – see Table 5.1, which contains data on spending across the categories for England in 2006/07). These data are compiled from returns submitted annually by PCTs and are subject to validation processes. Even at this aggregate level some interesting results emerge. It is not surprising that 'Problems of circulation' and 'Cancers and tumours' are ranked as the second- and third-highest spending areas respectively. However, it may be surprising to many to learn that 'Mental health disorders' is the area of highest expenditure, especially

Table 5.1: Programme budget categories and expenditure in 2006/07

Programme no	Programme name	£m	%
5	Mental health disorders	9,126	10.84
10	Problems of circulation	6,898	8.19
2	Cancers and tumours	4,352	5.17
13	Problems of the gastro-intestinal system	3,852	4.58
17	Problems of the genito-urinary system	3,755	4.46
11	Problems of the respiratory system	3,540	4.20
15	Problems of the musculoskeletal system	3,531	4.19
16	Problems due to trauma and injuries	2,992	3.55
7	Neurological	2,987	3.55
18	Maternity and reproductive health	2,932	3.48
12	Dental problems	2,644	3.14
6	Problems of learning disability	2,494	2.96
4	Endocrine, nutritional and metabolic problems	2,133	2.53
22	Social care needs	1,720	2.04
14	Problems of the skin	1,553	1.84
21	Healthy individuals	1,482	1.76
8	Problems of vision	1,382	1.64
1	Infectious diseases	1,301	1.55
3	Disorders of blood	1,035	1.23
19	Conditions of neonates	802	0.95
20	Adverse effects and poisoning	756	0.90
9	Problems of hearing	330	0.39
23	Other areas of spend/conditions		
a	*General medical services/personal medical services*	*7,257*	*8.62*
b	*Strategic health authorities (including WDCs)*	*3,514*	*4.17*
c	*National insurance contribution*	*0*	*0.00*
x	*Miscellaneous*	*11,825*	*14.05*
Total		**84,193**	**100.00**

given the regular characterisation of this area as the 'Cinderella' of health services. Currently, it appears that around £9 billion a year is being spent on this programme in England. An alternative reading of these data would be that most of the remaining NHS resources are being spent on physical health needs, although it is likely that mental health needs would also be addressed significantly within other programme areas. However, a natural first step might to ask how the £9 billion is currently being spent and whether this resource is being used to maximum effect for mental health patients before deciding whether to allocate more resources to the mental health pot.

At the local level, and referring back to Box 5.2, the starting point for programme budgeting is a retrospective appraisal of where health resources have been allocated. Now we know that this can be broken down into meaningful health programmes such as cancer, mental health and circulatory diseases for each PCT population. Objectives for each of these programmes can be set at the local level, incorporating national service frameworks and guidance from authoritative bodies such as NICE. It is then possible to look at the activity and outcomes generated by this investment and at the needs and inequalities that remain to be addressed so that adjustments in the following year's programme allocations can be made accordingly. Further national-level resources, such as the NHS National Knowledge Service (www.nks.nhs.uk), established by the inspirational Sir Muir Gray and summarising the evidence base in many areas of health care, can be drawn on in this process, requiring both managers and clinicians to work together to interpret such evidence for their local health economy.

Five years of PCT programme budget returns are now available on the Department of Health website (www.dh.gov.uk/Programme Budgeting). More recently, these returns have been linked to activity and outcomes data in interactive atlases published by the National Centre for Health Outcomes Development, which currently covers 15 programme budget categories. These are available to NHS users on the NHS intranet (nww.nchod.nhs.uk). Thus, it is now possible for commissioners of health care to link their programme objectives, activities and outcomes to estimates of expenditure, to compare these with their peer PCTs and to be more open and explicit about local needs and priorities.

As an example, Figure 5.2 provides data from an anonymised (but real) PCT showing its position against 30 similar PCTs on two attributes: expenditure per 100,000 population (adjusted for need) and health outcomes (see Figure 5.2 for definitions). 'Similar', here, is

—

defined by the Office for National Statistics (ONS), allowing PCTs to be clustered in the following way:

- regional cities
- centres with industry
- thriving London periphery
- London suburbs
- London centre
- London cosmopolitan
- prospering smaller towns
- new and growing towns
- prospering southern England
- coastal and countryside
- industrial hinterlands
- manufacturing towns.

This categorisation is useful, because, although the data set allows PCTs within strategic health authority boundaries to be compared with each other (or in any other way deemed necessary or useful), it may be more relevant to compare a PCT with others around the country that are similar in terms of rural–urban split, industrial heritage and so on.

Figure 5.2 is divided into four quadrants, which are derived by drawing a line perpendicular to each axis from the mid-rank 'score' (in this case, 15). Each quadrant is then labelled as shown, and the position of each programme category designated by its number and a corresponding diamond. The hollow diamonds along the top of the figure represent programme categories for which there are no outcome data as yet (the art and the science being works in progress). From the figure it can be seen that, in comparison with other PCTs in the ONS cluster group, this particular PCT's spend on substance abuse (programme category 5a) and poisoning (category 20) is comparatively high, but outcome data are unavailable; spend on respiratory system problems (category 11) is comparatively high and outcomes also rank comparatively highly; spend on maternity and reproductive health (category 18) is comparatively high but outcomes rank comparatively poorly; spend on cancers and tumours

Figure 5.2: Nowhere PCT: expenditure and outcomes rankings relative to ONS cluster groups

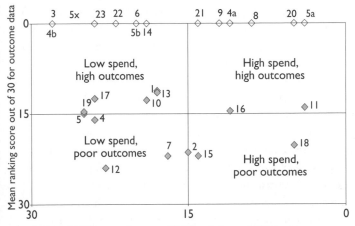

Ranking of PCT expenditure per 100,000 relative to ONS cluster group

KEY

Ranking of PCT expenditure per 100,000 population relative to ONS cluster group:
This is a ranking of PCT spend per 100,000 population for each programme category relative to all PCTs in the ONS cluster group (30 in total). 1 represents the highest spending PCT, 30 represents the lowest spending PCT in the cluster for each programme area.

Spend per 100,000 population indexed against the ONS cluster average:
This is a relative assessment of the proportional amount by which the PCT expenditure per 100,000 population is above or below the ONS cluster average for each programme category. A value of greater than 1 indicates the proportional amount that the PCT is spending above the ONS cluster average, whereas a value of less that 1 indicates the proportional amount that the PCT is spending under the ONS cluster average.

Mean ranking score out of 30 for outcome data:
This is the average score for the ranking of PCT outcome measures relative to the ONS cluster group (30 in total), for each programme category. Note that outcome data on prevalence was not used in the calculation of the mean score due to the ambiguous nature of a ranking based on high or low prevalence (however, it is reported for information). A mean ranking score of 1 indicates that the PCT on average ranked highest on the outcome measures compared with other PCTs in the ONS cluster group (that is, reports better outcomes than comparators). A mean ranking score of 30 indicates that the PCT on average ranked lowest on the outcome measures compared with other PCTs in the ONS cluster group (that is,

(category 2) ranks in the middle but outcomes rank comparatively poorly, with similar results for neurological systems problems (category 7) and musculoskeletal systems problems (category 15); spend on dental problems (category 12) is comparatively low but outcomes rank comparatively poorly, which may make it a candidate for more resources.

The main caveat of the data presented is that no inferences about causality between expenditure and outcomes can be drawn. The data are indicative of areas where further investigation at the local level might yield greater efficiencies in terms of improving outcomes gained for resources expended using the type of framework outlined in Boxes 5.2 and 5.3. The key is that these tools show commissioners where they might work with local clinicians, using more in-depth local data and evidence, in order to assess whether such programmes should receive more or fewer resources or remain at the current level.

Another key is that production of these data show that we can sensibly record resource use. Another indication of being able to conduct PBMA exercises is that, internationally, while the application of PBMA is not without its challenges, the framework has been used in well over 70 health organisations in Australia, New Zealand, Canada and the UK. One explanation for why it has not been used more widely may be, as Ruth McDonald (2002) has shown, that the NHS has a poor track record of adopting the outcomes of traditional economic evaluations other than at a national level, and that PBMA is perceived in a similar light. It is important to stress, however, that PBMA is different to economic evaluation in one crucial way. Although based on the same principles, PBMA uses these principles to create a *management process*, into which results from standard economic evaluations and other evidence can be incorporated; it is not simply expected that economic evaluations will be adopted, but the principles still can be. Indeed, it could be argued that such a process is the missing piece in the jigsaw of health care reform internationally, whereby defensible mechanisms are required to help health authorities remain within budget while balancing national guidance and local needs.

Conclusion

It is not surprising that record increases in expenditure in the UK NHS have coincided with unprecedented deficits. 'Crises' of this latter nature are not unfamiliar in other countries either. Ultimately, no one is really managing scarcity. Different parts of the organisations that make up publicly funded health care will deal separately with the different functions of finance, safety, quality and effectiveness, not recognising that these are all dependent on each other and that management processes need to be developed that take this message on board. Of course, one challenge not addressed yet is that of time. Readers who work in health care management may wonder how they can manage scarcity on top of everything else they doing. Without meaning to sound trite, there is one simple answer to this: drop what you are doing and get on with the most important job of all, that of managing scarce and precious publicly funded resources for maximum and equitable population health. More practically, the framework uses data that people already work with in their workplace.

One thing is certain – the status quo is not an option. In England, hospital providers are thinking of moving into the territory of primary care, as has happened in many parts of the US. The rhetoric of this sounds good; such integration of care would provide a seamless transition from the primary to the secondary sector and back again. But hospitals do not represent anyone. It could be argued that in the US no one is concerned with what is best for the overall population, as is the case with hospital providers in England. So this kind of integration is really about capturing more patients so as to protect the income of the acute sector. The only bodies with responsibility for assessing whether this is the way to go from a population perspective are (at least in England) PCTs and, it could be argued, national bodies such as NICE. What is needed to prevent hospital providers from simply taking over primary care in order to 'feed the beast' of the acute sector is an approach that can maximise population health with the resources available. The acute sector is not best placed to perform this task, and yet the market is currently rigged in its favour. I would argue that in England, a coalition of PCTs and NICE needs to take forward this agenda. I say this because they are the only two entities within the NHS in England that represent geographically defined populations, and if PCTs were much more involved in setting the NICE agenda, there would be less conflict between the two, resulting in a strong alliance against the cost-increasing tendencies of large acute hospitals and the pharmaceutical industry. It is up to you, as a concerned member of the public or a reader in some other (perhaps professional) role, to lobby our politicians to take on this agenda.

Although a counter-argument might be that it is politically challenging to work with explicit frameworks for managing scarce resources, surely it is better to have in place processes that can be used to defend particular decisions and are based on explicit criteria, and to manage these processes on a smaller scale, year on year, rather than suffer the periodic but drastic, embarrassing and non-evidence-based cuts of the sort currently faced by many organisations. Furthermore, having a health service that is not disproportionately dominated by the acute sector and is sustainable in terms of being publicly funded, crucially depends on getting to grips with managing scarcity.

Finally, it is a major indictment of those who legislate for and govern our health care systems that basic economics, as the 'science of scarcity', is not routinely taught to health care managers and clinicians (as well as medical doctors) who have to manage scarcity every day. Where does economics appear in the professional development agenda of these people? Indeed this is likely to be a crucial stage in the formal education of such professionals, as the notion of scarcity will be familiar to them, and they may think the only way out the dilemma (at least as far as their own small domain within the health care system is concerned) is to shout, scream and thump the table. As a recent editorial, by Richard Smith, in the *British Medical Journal* stated: 'Knowing nothing about economics leaves you almost as disadvantaged as somebody who is illiterate or knows nothing about history, science, or geography' (Smith, 2003). Having been introduced to the basics here, the more formal approaches to economic evaluation are outlined in Chapter Six, which will allow us to address the question that underlies all of the material presented so far: 'What's your health worth?'

Further reading

Gafni, A. and Birch, S. (1993) 'Guidelines for the adoption of new technologies: a prescription for uncontrolled growth in expenditures and how to avoid it', *Canadian Medical Association Journal*, vol 148, pp 913-17.

Ham, C. (2003) 'Improving the performance of health services: the role of clinical leadership', *Lancet*, vol 36, pp 1978-80.

McDonald, R. (2002) *Using Health Economics in Health Services: Rationing Rationally?* Buckingham: Open University Press.

Mitton, C. and Donaldson, C. (2004) *Priority Setting Toolkit: A Guide to the Use of Economics in Healthcare Decision Making*, London: BMJ Books.

Peacock, S., Ruta, D., Mitton, C., Donaldson, C., Bate, A. and Murtagh, M. (2006) 'Using economics for pragmatic and ethical priority setting: two checklists for doctors and managers', *British Medical Journal*, vol 332, pp 482-5.

Ruta, D., Donaldson, C. and Mitton, C. (2005) 'Programme budgeting and marginal analysis: a common resource management framework for doctors and managers?', *British Medical Journal*, vol 330, pp 1501-3.

Smith, R. (2003) 'What doctors and managers can learn from each other', *British Medical Journal*, vol 326, pp 610-11.

SIX

Economic evaluation

Introduction

The 'sustainability' question is frequently raised within the context of our publicly funded health care systems, and more and more new research directions are being taken to inform such a question. All clinical and public health areas need to seriously consider focusing on economic evaluation. This is the generic term for more commonly known methods of cost–effectiveness analysis (CEA) and cost–benefit analysis (CBA) and is based on the same principles as programme budgeting and marginal analysis.

Economic evaluation, in the formal sense described here, is now an accepted method of appraising health care programmes more generally. However, its use in evaluating interventions in many areas of clinical care is still rare, as my experience of writing introductory articles on economic evaluation for clinical journals specialising in different areas of clinical practice has shown. In one recent article, written with colleagues Jim Rankin and Helen Mason (Donaldson et al, 2007), a literature search of the CINAHL (1982-2006), MEDLINE (1966-2006), EMBASE (1980-2006) and Healthstar (1966-2006) electronic databases using the key search terms *economic evaluation, nurs$* and *orthop$* revealed only two studies. There was no indication in either study of a particularly sophisticated approach to economic evaluation and neither study related to orthopaedic nursing practice per se. The same is true of economic evaluation relating to liver disease, another area I have studied recently. It has to be said that this is a shocking state of affairs for two areas of care aimed at treating very common conditions. One reason for the lack of formal economic evaluation in the literature may be due to the lack of understanding of basic principles involved in doing this type of research. This chapter tries to rectify the situation to some extent, as well as demonstrating (if Chapter Five did not succeed) that application of the basic principles of economic evaluation in health care is entirely ethical, and, indeed, that failing to apply these principles is both unprofessional and unethical.

We will not dwell on these principles for long; they are the same as those outlined in Chapter Five, which discussed the constant, and natural, tension between what the public purse can afford and what people would like health services to do, health economic evaluation being about how scarce health care resources are used to produce the greatest benefit to the community. Without scarcity, anyone could have as much of anything they want and there would be no need for economics, or, for that matter, economists. This leads to the concept of opportunity cost. By using resources in one activity, we give up the opportunity of using them in some other way. The opportunity cost is the benefit that would have been obtained from those resources in their next best alternative use. When concerned about the cost of a service, it is not parsimony that feeds our interest, but the health benefits that could be gained by using those resources in a different way. In any area of clinical care, I am sure an honest assessment by many health professionals would lead them to admit that, if resources could be reallocated in some way, greater overall gain to patients might result, at least potentially. If so, other things being equal, that change should be made. The logical conclusion to this is that it is necessary to know what benefits and resources used in alternative courses of action could be funded by our limited budgets. It is only by knowing this that decisions on the best combinations of resources to maximise patient and public health can be made.

The implications of these principles are outlined in the following sections. The starting point is a very basic summary of what we mean by costs and benefits in health care, which will lead us into describing a highly useful decision matrix, showing how costs and benefits can be brought together to make decisions. From there, we move on to the challenges and important subtleties of economic evaluation. These centre mainly around how 'health' and other important contributions of health care to the welfare of society are measured and valued, setting up the question 'What's your health worth?' for Chapter Seven. As with most activity, there is more to

—

economic evaluation than meets the eye. A detailed description of all the methodological issues involved in performing an economic evaluation is beyond the scope of this book. An article written with a colleague Phil Shackley (1997) provides more detail on such issues, while Mike Drummond and colleagues' (2005) seminal work is a more popular 'how to' text on economic evaluation. Both are listed in the further reading section at the end of the chapter.

From principles to decisions

A very general classification of what economists mean by costs and benefits is given in Table 6.1. The approach is usually broad (societal) rather than one that focuses on publicly funded health resources or resource use. Resources used are measured in money, usually referred to as costs. However, it is important to remember that this 'money' is not the sort that can be accrued in a bank; it provides a measure of different packages of resources in a common unit through which the health (and other) benefits associated with these alternative packages can be compared. Remember, only by having information on costs and benefits can the combination of health care activities be chosen that maximises benefit to the community from our limited budget. Also, as demonstrated in Chapter Five, this often involves analysing

Table 6.1: Costs and outcomes considered for inclusion in an economic evaluation

Costs	Benefits/outcomes
Costs to health care system Staffing Consumables Overheads Capital	Health gains (in terms of life expectancy, quality of life or both) Health deterioration (for example, side effects, anxiety)
Other public sector costs Community services Ambulance services	Non-health-related effects on well-being (for example, pregnant women may have preferences over the location for delivery of their baby)
Costs incurred by clients and family Inputs to treatment Out-of-pocket expenses Time lost from work	Changes in production due to illness and treatment (could be either gains or losses)

the optimal nature and extent of activities rather than whether they should take place at all.

Basically, in making service delivery choices and setting health care priorities, we want to maximise benefits and minimise opportunity costs. To achieve this level of efficiency, we need to be able to link inputs to outputs, or costs to benefits, for the different courses of action making claims on our scarce resources.

The 'evidence-based medicine' movement has promoted the use of randomised trials, other controlled comparisons and systematic reviews of effectiveness as methods to compare what works (that is, what improves health) when examining alternative ways to treat similar groups of patients. However, although useful, 'what works' is not enough. If 'value for money' is the goal, this means combining information on what works (or 'effectiveness') with costs. More often than not, a new proposal for treatment is compared with current practice. Linking effectiveness to costs will then allow us to determine whether a new procedure is:

- less costly and at least as effective as its comparator (the status quo), in which case the new procedure would be judged, unequivocally, to be a better use of health care resources (in economics language, dominant and, referring back to Chapter Five, 'more technically efficient'); or
- more costly, and more effective, than the comparator, in which case a judgement would have to be made about whether the extra cost of the new procedure is worth incurring given the gains in health achieved (an 'allocative efficiency' question).

The allocative efficiency question also takes us back to Chapter Five and the notion of opportunity cost. Given that a new procedure is more beneficial but is going to cost more than current practice, should more resources be allocated to that area of care given the alternative uses of the resources available? Remember the example of hips versus hearts in Chapter Five. Expanding resources in one of these programmes may mean a necessary contraction in the other. As will be seen below, a lot of economic evaluation, as currently applied in health care, fails to recognise this fundamental point.

—

For now, data on effectiveness and costs can be brought together in a matrix format (Figure 6.1) to help judge whether a new procedure is preferable to the status quo. In Figure 6.1, it can be seen that, relative to the status quo, the new procedure could achieve (1) greater effectiveness, (2) the same level of effectiveness or (3) less effectiveness. Of course, a fourth option is possible whereby, after reviewing the literature, there is not enough evidence to make a judgement on whether the new procedure is more or less effective. Within evaluations based on randomised trials and other controlled comparisons, for example, the main aim is to identify data on the relative effectiveness of health care interventions. The use of systematic review, promoted most prominently by bodies such as the Cochrane Collaboration and using techniques like meta-analysis, also has the identification and promulgation of evidence on effectiveness as its primary goal.

Figure 6.1: Matrix linking effectiveness with cost

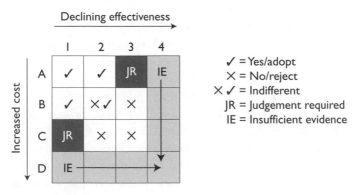

Effectiveness
Compared with the control treatment, the experimental treatment has:
1. Evidence of greater effectiveness
2. Evidence of no difference in effectiveness
3. Evidence of less effectiveness
4. Not enough evidence of effectiveness

Cost
Compared with the control treatment, the experimental treatment has:
A. Evidence of cost savings
B. Evidence of no difference in costs
C. Evidence of greater costs
D. Not enough evidence on costs

What economics most obviously adds to the evaluation is consideration of the resource consequences of any proposed changes in the way health care is delivered. Thus, in terms of cost, a new procedure could (A) save costs, (B) result in no difference in costs or (C) increase costs. (Again, there is the possibility of there being not enough evidence to judge, as represented by row D.)

Figure 6.1 is adapted from that which appeared in early editions of the Cochrane Collaboration Handbook (www.cochrane-handbook. org) and in a book I co-edited on evidence-based health economics with Miranda Mugford and Luke Vale. For any procedure, the optimum position on the matrix (Figure 6.1) is square A1, where an experimental treatment would both save costs and have greater effectiveness relative to current treatment. In squares A1, A2 and B1, the new procedure is more efficient and is assigned a ✓ response to the question of whether it is to be preferred to current practice. In squares B3, C2, and C3, the new procedure is less efficient and thus receives a ✕ response. In squares A3 and C1, a judgement would be required as to whether the more costly procedure is worthwhile in terms of the additional effectiveness gained (the allocative efficiency question again). Square B2 is neutral, as there is no difference in either costs or effectiveness. All the grey areas in the matrix represent situations in which there is not enough evidence on effectiveness, costs or either to judge whether the new procedure is to be preferred.

Generally, cells A1, A2 and B1 (as well as B3, C2 and C3) represent three types of situation addressed by CEA. Here, CEA tells us how to achieve a given outcome at less cost or how to spend a limited amount of funds more effectively. There may be situations where effectiveness is measured in multidimensional terms, in which case a composite assessment of the value of these outcomes, in the form of quality adjusted life years (QALYs) or even willingness to pay (WTP), may be useful. QALYs and WTP are explained in more detail below.

In situations represented by cells A3 and C1, the question of the additional cost of achieving the health gains becomes important. It is also useful here to have effectiveness gains valued in terms of QALYs or WTP. An incremental value of the benefits gained can then be calculated along with an incremental value of the cost incurred to achieve such a gain. Ideally, with the benefits valued in such a manner, it would be possible for decision makers to compare the benefits gained by the new procedure with those that would be gained by some alternative uses of the incremental resources the new procedure would require. Thus, once again, the opportunity cost of the new procedure would be highlighted. Cost–utility and cost–benefit analyses are designed for these types of question, the former using QALYs and the latter usually making use of monetary valuation of benefits such as WTP.

Thus there are two additional contributions that economic evaluation can make to systematic reviews of effectiveness. First, the matrix in Figure 6.1 shows that the economic approach adds the consideration of resource use to effectiveness evidence. By highlighting issues of technical efficiency and opportunity cost, this alone should make evidence-based medicine more relevant for decision making. It is my belief that one of the most important things clinicians can do is to categorise all interventions within their specialty according to the matrix in Figure 6.1. They can then ask themselves why they are not doing more of the procedures in cells A1, A2 and B1, and, if they are doing them, why are they continuing with procedures in cells B3, C2 and C3. Judgements about cells A3 and C1 are more tricky, but more sophisticated tools of economic evaluation may be able to help. Thus, and second, although disaggregated outcomes are of use for clinical and patient information, composite measures of the benefits of health care, in the form of QALYs or WTP, may further aid the decision-making process for resource allocation decisions.

Quality adjusted life years

The QALY is a health outcome measure that considers both quality and quantity of life over some period of time. The quantity component of the QALY is simply the number of life years under consideration. This can represent the number of life years saved, which would be the extension of an individual's life, measured in years, due to a particular course of treatment. Alternatively, quantity of life can be a measure of a specific time span during an individual's life, say, when an individual has a non-life threatening illness that lasts for some period of time.

The quality component of the QALY, or quality adjustment for each life year under consideration, can be derived through a number of different methods. In each case, a measure between 0 and 1 is derived, with 0 generally being equated with death and 1 with full health. Different states of health, lying between these two anchor states, are assigned values between 0 and 1 depending on their severity. The methods for deriving these scores, which are often referred to as utilities or health state valuations, are described below.

Once an index or quality adjustment score has been obtained, the number of years under consideration is multiplied by the index score to derive the QALY. The QALY is illustrated in Figures 6.2a and 6.2b. These figures illustrate the QALY gain (the dark shaded area) of kidney transplant over dialysis in treating chronic renal failure. Year zero in each figure represents the point at which a patient is treated. In both figures, transplant, on average, will increase patient survival by seven years (from 13 years to 20 years) over and above dialysis. However, dialysis also reduces quality of life relative to transplant, as seen on the vertical axis. In Figure 6.2a, it is assumed that transplant leads to a full quality of life (valued at 1.0) while dialysis involves a degree of impairment (with quality of life valued at 0.8). This means that, although transplant confers a seven-year survival advantage, it brings about a gain of 9.6 QALYs over dialysis – the 9.6 being made up of a 0.2 gain (that is, 1.0 instead of 0.8 quality of life) for 13 years (for $0.2 \times 13 = 2.6$ QALYs) plus seven extra years in full health (or seven QALYs), for a total of 9.6 QALYs. If the degree of impairment under dialysis is worse, say 0.6, the QALY gain from transplant is even greater, at 12.2 (see Figure 6.2b). This example has been included to show how important it is to actually measure the quality of life aspect, as, in this example, it makes a difference to the QALY gains whether life on dialysis is rated at 0.6 or 0.8.

Before moving on to discuss how such measurement is undertaken, two other points are worth noting. First, the idea is that estimates of QALY gains are combined with costs. Therefore, taking the QALY gains expressed in Figure 6.2a, if transplant resulted in a net saving of resources, a 'dominant' situation would arise whereby transplant leads to greater QALYs and cost savings – an unambiguous improvement in efficiency. However, if transplant were to cost, say, £96,000 more

—

Figure 6.2a: Assessing the QALY gain from transplant

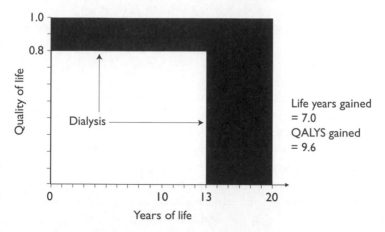

Life years gained
= 7.0
QALYS gained
= 9.6

Figure 6.2b: Assessing the QALY gain from transplant

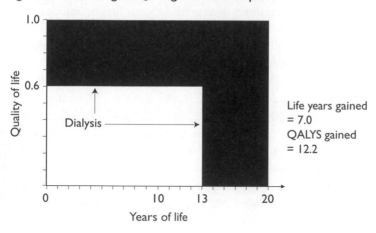

Life years gained
= 7.0
QALYS gained
= 12.2

than dialysis, this would result in an incremental cost per QALY of £10,000. This might appear to be good value for money, but would actually depend on how many QALYs could be generated by using this money elsewhere, either in chronic renal failure or in treating a completely different set of patients elsewhere in the health care system. This is a controversial statement, as it assumes that QALYs are comparable across disparate groups of people and conditions, although it could be argued that this position has to be accepted, given the scarcity of resources and the need to make choices.

There are two main types of QALY: generic and condition-specific.

Generic QALYs

Generic QALYs can be applied to any group of interest and are typically based on scores from the general public. For example, patients in a given study could be asked to complete a questionnaire in which they rate themselves in terms of different dimensions of health. The responses on these dimensions correspond to health states that can be scored. These scores, or utilities, are usually obtained through a survey of the general public in which participants are given a description of the health states and are asked to rate the states between 0 = death and 1 = full health. As described above, the scores, which correspond to the health state indicated by the patients under study through the questionnaire, can then be multiplied by the relevant length of life to derive the QALY.

One of the most widely used tools for measuring generic QALYs is EQ-5D, which was devised and developed by the EuroQol Group (1990). The five dimensions of the EQ-5D are mobility, self-care, usual activities, pain/discomfort and anxiety/depression. Each dimension has three levels, as outlined in Box 6.1, thus enabling the EQ-5D to define 243 different health states. The inclusion of two extra health states, unconscious and dead, means there are 245 possible health state descriptions.

The EQ-5D is designed to be administered in the form of a self-completed questionnaire. Subjects are asked to define their own health state in terms of the five dimensions and their levels, and then are asked to mark on a visual analogue scale how good or bad they think their current health is. Based on the time trade-off technique (described below), a tariff of quality of life scores for each EQ-5D health state has been developed in several countries. The tariff allows each of the EQ-5D health states, identifiable by a unique five-digit number corresponding to the levels for each of the five dimensions, to be converted into a score that can be used as the quality adjustment weight in the calculation of QALYs. Scores based on UK and North

Box 6.1: Dimensions of the EuroQol EQ-5D

Mobility
- I have no problems in walking about
- I have some problems in walking about
- I am confined to bed

Self-care
- I have no problems with self-care
- I have some problems washing or dressing myself
- I am unable to wash or dress myself

Usual activities (for example, work, study, housework, family or leisure activities)
- I have no problems with performing my usual activities
- I have some problems with performing my usual activities
- I am unable to perform my usual activities

Pain/discomfort
- I have no pain or discomfort
- I have moderate pain or discomfort
- I have extreme pain or discomfort

Anxiety/depression
- I am not anxious or depressed
- I am moderately anxious or depressed
- I am extremely anxious or depressed

American samples have been derived by the Measurement and Valuation of Health Group (by Paul Dolan and colleagues, 1995) and Jeff Johnson and colleagues respectively.

These measures have been criticised for being too simplistic and insensitive to changes in health status. However, measures such as EQ-5D and the Health Utilities Index (devised in Canada) remain very popular.

Condition-specific QALYs

In the case of condition-specific QALYs, the health state descriptions provided to the subjects under study focus directly on the characteristics of the condition being evaluated. There are two main methods of generating condition-specific QALYs: standard gamble and time trade-off. The standard gamble is based directly on the axioms of standard utility theory and is the classic method of measuring preferences under uncertainty. The technique can be used to measure health state preferences for chronic and temporary health states, although the discussion here focuses on the use of the technique to calculate QALYs for a chronic health state preferred to death.

An example of the standard gamble is shown in Figure 6.3. To measure preferences for health state i, subjects are asked to choose between two alternatives. One offers the certain outcome of remaining in the chronic health state for the rest of one's life, while the other is a gamble representing a treatment with two possible outcomes. These two outcomes are to return to full health for the rest of one's life, with an associated probability p of occurring, or immediate death, which has a probability of occurrence of $1 - p$. The probability p of a successful outcome is varied by an iterative process until the subject is indifferent when faced with the choice between the gamble and the certainty. The probability at which the subject is indifferent is taken as the utility value of the health state, which can be used to calculate the QALY. A practical example of this for the state 'being on dialysis' is provided in Figure 6.4. In surveys of patients or the general public, the health state 'being on dialysis' would be described in more detail to respondents, but is used here

Figure 6.3: Standard gamble for a chronic health state preferred to death

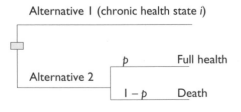

Alternative 1 (chronic health state *i*)

Alternative 2

p — Full health

$1 - p$ — Death

merely for illustrative purposes and to be able to relate to the example displayed in Figure 6.2b.

Time trade-off was developed by George Torrance and colleagues (1986) at McMaster University in Ontario as a substitute for the standard gamble technique. The intention was to develop a technique specifically for use in health care, which gave the same (or similar) values as the standard gamble but was easier for subjects to understand. Two important differences between time trade-off and the standard gamble should be noted. First, time trade-off does not have an axiomatic foundation, and second, subjects are asked to choose between two certain alternatives rather than between a certain outcome and a gamble. Like the standard gamble, time trade-off can

Figure 6.4: Standard gamble of certainty of 'being on dialysis' versus uncertain treatment involving full health or death

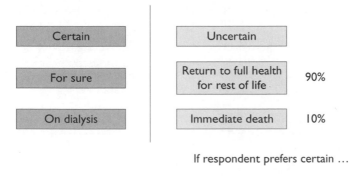

If respondent prefers certain ...

... adjust the chances appropriately (by making the 'uncertain' treatment more attractive), for example

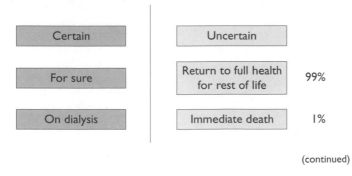

(continued)

Figure 6.4 (continued)

On the other hand, suppose that when presented with …

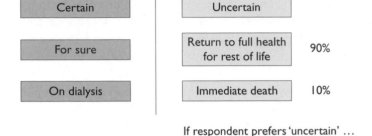

If respondent prefers 'uncertain' …

… adjust the chances to make 'uncertain' less attractive

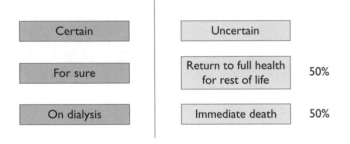

If after series of such alterations to probabilities, respondent settles on equivalence of scenarios as follows …

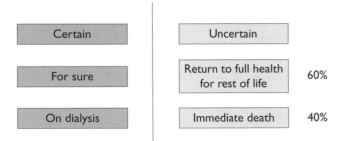

Quality adjustment index assigned = 0.6

be used to elicit health state preferences for chronic and temporary health states that may or may not be preferred to death.

An example of the time trade-off approach for a chronic health state preferred to death is shown in Figure 6.5. Preferences for health state i are established by eliciting from subjects the number of years in full health (Z years) that is equivalent to spending the rest of their life (T years) in the chronic health state. The value at which the subject is indifferent when faced with a choice between the two alternatives is taken as the value of the health state, which can then be used to calculate the number of QALYs from the treatment in the same way as for the standard gamble.

Figure 6.5: Time trade-off for a chronic health state preferred to death

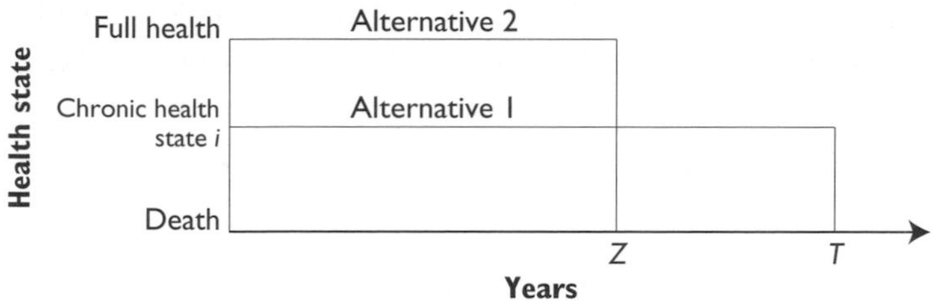

Willingness to pay

The most common method of measuring health care benefits in CBA is WTP. The principle of WTP is fairly simple – the utility that an individual gains from something like a hip replacement is valued by the maximum amount that he or she would be willing to pay for that new hip. With this technique, individuals are given a description of a health state, or different types of health care, and are asked, hypothetically, how much they would be willing to pay for that state or type of care. Depending on the context, information may also be given on the risk of ever needing such care in the first place. WTP can be used in the context of questions pertaining to both allocative and technical efficiency.

The technique of WTP is often criticised for attempting to assign a monetary value to things that are considered by many to be incommensurate with monetary valuation, such as the environment, human life and so on. However, it has to be remembered that such valuations are being made, often implicitly, anyway. Whenever a decision is made to spend money or deny care a value of life or health is implied. What is important is not the unit of value per se, but rather the notion of sacrifice embodied in the WTP technique. In valuing a health care programme, it is difficult to ask respondents what services they would give up to have more of that programme. It is easier to ask individuals to state the maximum amount they would be willing to pay for more of the programme and for some possible alternative uses of those resources. Thus, it is largely for convenience of comparison that money is the chosen numeraire.

One key advantage of WTP over other measures of benefit such as the QALY is that it provides the opportunity for individuals to value other potential benefits of health care beyond just health gain. One of the assumptions of QALYs is that the only benefit from health care is improvement in health-related quality of life and/or survival. However, there is evidence that this is not always the case, as shown by classic pieces of work by Berwick and Weinstein (1985), and Mooney and Lange (1993). Other possible sources of benefit may include the provision of information (for example, from screening), dignity (for example, in long-term care), autonomy (for example, in community care) and the process of care (for example, invasive versus non-invasive interventions).

Depending on the context of the evaluation, there are a number of different ways in which individuals can be asked about their WTP. These include out-of-pocket payments, one-off extra taxation payments and payments for insurance. There are also a number of different ways of asking WTP questions. These include payment card questions, in which subjects are presented with a series of prompts from which to select a value; open-ended questions, in which respondents are asked to state their maximum WTP without prompting; and closed-ended questions, in which each respondent is presented with a WTP value (varied across respondents) and asked to indicate whether or not they would be prepared to pay that value. All of these methods have advantages and disadvantages.

Although WTP does define benefit more broadly than QALYs, a frequent criticism is that WTP is inevitably a function of ability to pay, which, it is argued, could have implications for equity. My own work has shown that this can be dealt with, however, by weighting the WTP values. It is also worth noting that QALYs suffer from a similar problem, with attempts to add in wider considerations having been led by people like Erik Nord (1999) in Norway. These issues stem from the fact that all such measures are proxies for utility because utility itself cannot be measured directly.

Lastly, in cases where the total WTP elicited from users of a programme is greater than the programme cost, it may be tempting to conclude that such a programme is worthwhile. However, the opportunity cost context is one where resources for such a programme will have to come from some other use. In determining 'worthwhileness', the relevant set of values are those of the broader community, as opposed to the individual users of the service, as the question is one of allocative efficiency. In recognising this, much of my own work with Jan Abel Olsen (1998) from the University of Tromso has involved asking samples of members of the public about their relative WTP for quite disparate health care options that are characterised as competing for money from the limited taxation pot. That said, the WTP values of the users of the services being evaluated are still useful in that context. For instance, such values could indicate that the preferences of a minority group are particularly strong. If this strength of preference is not sufficient to outweigh that of the majority, such values may still indicate to the decision maker that providing both types of care being evaluated is the fairest option. Of course, it should be remembered that providing such choice might come at a substantial cost.

Appraising the economic appraisal

Critical appraisal of economic evaluations is as important as appraisal of any other piece of research. Full guides to critical appraisal are provided in many health economics publications. This includes assessment of standard items that should be asked on any piece of research, such as whether the study question is clear and relevant and whether the conclusions drawn by the authors are warranted from the results reported. More specifically, the main questions should concern the costs and benefits that have been included, any key aspect that is missing, and whether the costs and benefits have been measured and valued appropriately. With respect to the notion of value that underlies this book, however, three further aspects are worth discussing in a little more detail, as all are controversial: time, equity and the dreaded incremental cost–effectiveness ratio.

Time and discounting: is an ounce of prevention really worth a pound of cure?

Not all costs and benefits of health care programmes occur at the same point in time. The most obvious example is that of prevention, where costs are incurred early for the achievement of benefits (and cost savings) at a later date. The question then arises as to whether costs and benefits arising at different points in time should be given equal weighting. Most economists would say they should not, because individuals in society display a tendency to prefer to put off costs to the future rather than pay them now.

This 'time preference' arises because of the opportunity costs that would arise by allocating funds to pay costs now rather than having them available to pursue some other beneficial activity in the meantime. A cost arising in the future impinges on us less than a cost of equivalent magnitude arising today and so is 'discounted'. For example, most of us are familiar with the concept of a credit card, which shows a preference to put off costs to the future and for even paying a premium (in the form of interest payments) to do so. Part of the interest payment reflects the opportunity costs to the lender of not having these funds available to pursue some other beneficial activity in the meantime.

The same argument applies to valuation of the benefits of health care. Benefits occurring now are generally thought to be of greater value to us than a benefit of the same magnitude that arises in the future. Of course, to treat health gains in this way is controversial, a classic debate having taken place in health economics between Cairns, on one hand, and Parsonage and Neuberger, on the other, in 1992. By introducing a discount rate, future QALYs will be lower than if there were no discount rate when looked at from the perspective of the current day. The discount rate that is used should reflect the rate at which society prefers to trade off benefits (and costs) occurring sooner rather than later. For example, at present the UK Treasury is recommending a discount rate of 3.5% per annum for both costs and benefits and most other governments have also made such recommendations.

As such, rates are compounded from year to year, and, all else being equal, discounting can count quite severely against prevention and public health interventions for which health benefits may not arise until some time quite far into the future.

Implications for equity

Health economists are often accused of being too concerned with maximising things (for example, maximising health from available resources) without paying due concern to issues of equity. However, it should be remembered that concerns for equity also arise from scarcity of resources; otherwise, it would be considered 'fair' for people to use as much of any resource (including health care) as they wish. This means that costs and benefits still need to be measured. A concern for equity requires us to provide data on *who* accrues the benefits and incurs the costs of resource allocation decisions, in addition to the magnitude of such costs and benefits. It is only by estimating the costs and benefits of proposed changes of action that decisions can be made to produce a more equitable and efficient use of resources.

The equity question raises the issue of 'weights' to attach to health gains for different beneficiaries of care. To put this another way, a common argument in relation to elderly people who are major beneficiaries of many health services is that, on the one hand, they should be given less priority, as they have already consumed their 'fair share' of resources. On the other hand, it is argued that if they are older, they are likely to present for treatment with more severe conditions (so other things are not now equal) and therefore are more deserving of intervention. At the other end of the age spectrum, should health gains to children be weighted higher than for other members of the population, and, if so, are we talking about fully grown children (say, 5- to 10-year-olds), newborns or both? Introducing other aspects, should 'culpability' count whereby an individual's past lifestyle might weigh for or against them when being considered for treatment? Or is it the case that an individual's past lifestyle is determined more by social conditions than by their own actions, in which case there is less blame to be attached to people in ill health?

These questions have spawned much research in recent years by health economists and others. Unfortunately, these issues are, as yet, unresolved in policy circles. Experts may say things like 'gains to children are worth more' and 'people in more severe health states should be given priority', but, as yet, no government has explicitly adopted policies on issues such as these. Likewise, although members of the public may make similar pronouncements, they will often react in the opposite way when faced with a possible policy change on such bases. The most famous example of this, reported by the well-known US economist John Graham (2003), is the abandoned attempt by the US Environmental Protection Agency to instigate a 'senior health discount' on older lives saved from environmental regulation (e.g. for clean air), whereby such lives would be valued at two thirds the rate of others. When trying to 'sell' such a notion on a road trip around the US, members of the public objected so much that it was dropped, despite the fact that the idea came from results of surveys of members of the public in the first place.

Beware the incremental cost-effectiveness ratio

The ratio of incremental QALYs gained to incremental costs incurred, referred to earlier in the chapter, is commonly known as the ICER (or incremental cost-effectiveness ratio). I have not used that term because I do not like it, for reasons I briefly explain below. Ultimately, however, it raises an important question, which will be addressed in Chapter Eight.

First, the ICER has little to do with cost-effectiveness as defined above. Usually the intervention for which the ICER is calculated is compared with current practice. As resources are already committed to current practice, the *incremental* costs involved mean that more resources would have to be allocated to the programme of care in which the evaluated intervention resides. In a cash-limited health care system, this means that these resources would have to come from other competing areas of care. This is an allocative efficiency consideration, and that is not what cost-effectiveness is about. Declaring something as 'cost-effective' gives the impression to decision makers not only that it should be implemented, but also that this can be done at no cost. However, there will be a cost if other competing areas lose out.

Furthermore, health technology assessment (HTA) agencies tend to treat all ICERs in the same way. Thus, a respiratory therapy with a low ICER (or, say, £5,000 per QALY) that improves health-related quality of life alone would tend to be declared 'cost-effective' regardless of how many people will gain. If a large proportion of the population were to gain from such a therapy, the opportunity cost of its adoption could be large, and perhaps unaffordable. Likewise, a high ICER for treatment for a rare, serious condition, such as surgery for neuroblastoma (at, say, £120,000 per QALY) is likely to be declared by most health economists as 'not cost-effective', even although its total cost to society is likely to be minimal. Is each of these situations the same? Cost per QALY calculations would imply the latter be discontinued, but society, by continuing to conduct surgeries for neuroblastoma, says not. This raises serious questions about the notion of the QALY and the state of health economic evaluation.

What health economists need to do is, first, be consistent in terms of the definitions of things like CEA and CBA and how they are applied in practice. A simple way round this is to ban the term 'ICER' from our language. Why not use the term 'incremental cost per QALY', as that is what it is? Economists also need to be more honest in recognising that anything of this incremental nature has major allocative efficiency implications. When a health economist declares something as 'cost-effective', you need to think about whether this was based on an incremental analysis, and, if so, who or what might lose out as a result. Decision makers, too, need to get smarter in their understanding of these economic notions and face up to the tough allocative efficiency questions; stop doing things that provide little (though some) health return for resources invested because other uses of the resources would be better for society in toto.

One further issue of interest that the incremental cost per QALY raises is what should society be paying for an extra QALY anyway. There is no accepted global standard and even individual countries have not declared such a value. The only exception to this is the UK where a range of £20,000-30,000 per QALY, above which an intervention is less likely to be approved for use in the NHS in England, was declared by Michael Rawlins and Tony Culyer in their classic article in the *British Medical Journal*. They should know; they were chair and vice-chair of National Institute for Health and Clinical Excellence (NICE) at the time, the value having been arrived at through expert judgement of health economists and others at NICE's inception in 1999.

There are different ways one can think of how to arrive at a value. One is to accept that the health care budget in most countries is decided on an annual basis by parliament. To then maximise QALYs produced by that budget, the investment and disinvestment decisions made by health authorities (or primary care trusts in the UK) can then be examined in order to establish the cost per QALY at the margin at which such entities appear to be operating. This would aid the search for a value, as, for example, if the disinvestments made by these authorities were to have a lower cost per QALY gained than the recommendations made by a national HTA agency, such as NICE, this could be taken as evidence that the NICE 'threshold' is too high.

Unfortunately, this idea would seem to be rather far-fetched at the moment. To date, in various publicly funded health care systems, no systematic framework for commissioning, which recognises scarcity and can explicitly address trade-offs, has been implemented. I know this as a health economist who has done more than most in terms of working globally with heath organisations to try to improve their decision-making processes. It would seem that the development of frameworks, such as programme budgeting and marginal analysis (see Chapter Five), is essential for matching national priorities with local needs and to provide local health organisations with a defensible mechanism for (occasionally) justifying a focus on the local as well as the national agenda. When in place, perhaps the system could iterate towards the value of a QALY at the margin. However, only a few years ago in the UK, the Health Committee of the House of Commons stated that practical systems and structures should be put in place to improve capacity to implement guidance, as implicit prioritisation was insufficient. The committee stated that the government must work towards 'a comprehensive framework for health care prioritisation, underpinned by an explicit set of ethical and rational values to allow the relative costs and benefits of different areas of NHS spending to be comparatively assessed in an informed way' (see House of Commons Health Committee, Second Report of Session 2001-2, National Institute for Clinical Excellence, HC 515-1).

More recent assessment of primary care trusts, through the World Class Commissioning initiative in England, would seem to show little movement towards this ideal. UK-based health economists, John Appleby, Nancy Devlin and Dave Parkin, in their recent and admirable study, state that 'a definitive finding about the consistency or otherwise of NICE and NHS cost-effectiveness thresholds would require very many decisions to be observed, combined with a detailed understanding of the local decision making processes.' The most rigorous valuations to date are those of Steve Martin, Nigel Rice and Pete Smith (2008), who attempted to estimate what it costs the NHS in England to produce a QALY in the areas of cancer and circulatory disease, arriving at values of £11,960 and £19,070 respectively. However, these are for only two of the 23 disease categories within the English NHS programme budgeting data set used as the basis for these estimations. Values are likely to vary widely once estimated for all, if indeed such estimation is possible. It is also well known that valuations for other conditions, such as heroic treatment for neuroblastoma, mentioned above, come out very high, while those for other (respiratory) conditions are quite low (at around £5,000). Identification of such a range is useful, but it is not clear how much further, compared with other approaches, it gets us towards validating or querying the NICE threshold.

A complementary activity to such searches is to bring together the QALY and WTP approaches outlined above to survey members of the public about their WTP for different types of health gain. Assuming survey respondents think of publicly funded health care as being at full efficiency and unable to provide more services (or more QALYs) without extra payments being made, expressed WTP amounts would be a reasonable representation of a value of a QALY at the margin. This may then reasonably approximate what an individual budget-holder, like a health authority, may say is the value (if health authorities used QALYs and if they behaved in an economically rational and QALY-maximising fashion). Other potential uses of such an approach are twofold. First, any resulting value would place an upper limit on what health care spending on a QALY would be, as hypothetical responses by members of the public to such emotive questions are likely to be at the upper end of value. Second, if no single value exists, because things like life-saving QALYs are valued differently to those that improve quality of life, the most legitimate group to determine this is, in my view, the public, whose tax monies are being spent by publicly funded health care.

Conclusion

The practice of economic evaluation may not be straightforward, but its logic is simple. In the real world of patient care and public health interventions, the application of economic principles is required. Otherwise, in a cash-limited system, any amount of (effective) care should be provided to any patient with no limits placed on the amount of (effective) care given up by others. Thus, the measurement of costs and benefits has both an ethical and practical contribution to make to designing health services to best meet the needs of the community.

Economic evaluations contribute to the future sustainability of publicly funded health services, as, by definition, they ensure that we get the best out of such services. If such analyses are conducted on a widespread basis, they can be used to illustrate to governments what is being sacrificed by making cuts to services. Given the scarcity of health economists themselves and the tendency of health economists not to devote themselves to just one area of clinical practice, there would be an obvious role for health professionals in working with economists to design and implement such evaluations in any field of clinical practice. At the very least, it should be an ethical imperative for clinicians to classify care in their area of practice, using best evidence, according to the matrix in Figure 6.1.

—

Beyond this, QALYs and WTP can prove very useful. However, as the inaugural chair of NICE, Sir Michael Rawlins, has stated on many occasions, these are 'tools not rules' for decision making. You have been told what to look out for when the health economist comes with declarations of 'cost-effectiveness'. Now we can progress to the question, 'What is your health worth?'

Further reading

Appleby, J., Devlin, N., Parkin, D. et al (2009) 'Searching for cost effectiveness thresholds in the NHS', *Health Policy*, 91, pp 239–45.

Berwick, D.M. and Weinstein, M.C. (1985) 'What do patients value? Willingness to pay for ultrasound in normal pregnancy?', *Medical Care*, vol 23, pp 881-93.

Cairns, J. (1992) 'Discounting and health benefits: another perspective', *Health Economics*, vol 1, pp 76-9.

Dolan, P., Gudex, C., Kind, P. and Williams, A. (1995) *A Social Tariff for the EuroQol: Results from a UK General Population Survey*, Centre for Health Economics Discussion Paper 138, York: Centre for Health Economics, University of York.

Donaldson, C. (1999) 'Valuing the benefits of publicly-provided healthcare: does "ability to pay" preclude the use of "willingness to pay"?', *Social Science and Medicine*, vol 49, pp 551-63.

Donaldson, C., Mason, H. and Rankin, J.A. (2007) 'Economic evaluation and orthopaedic nursing', *Journal of Orthopaedic Nursing*, vol 11, pp 113-21.

Donaldson, C., Mugford, M. and Vale, L. (eds) (2002) *Evidence-based Health Economics: From Effectiveness to Efficiency in Systematic Review.* London: BMJ Books.

Donaldson, C. and Shackley, P. (1997) 'Economic evaluation', in R. Detels, W.W. Holland, J. McEwen and G.S. Omenn (eds) *Oxford Textbook of Public Health (Third Edition) Volume 2: The Methods of Public Health*, Oxford: Oxford University Press, pp 849-71.

Drummond, M.F., Sculpher M., O'Brien, B., Stoddart, G. and
Torrance, G. (2005) *Methods for the Economic Evaluation of
Healthcare Programmes* (3rd edn), Oxford: Oxford University
Press.
EuroQol Group (1990) 'EuroQol – a new facility for the
measurement of health-related quality of life', *Health Policy*,
vol 16, pp 199-208.
Graham, J.D. (2003) 'Memorandum to the President's
Management Council, benefit-cost methods and lifesaving
rules', Office of Information and Regulatory Affairs, Office of
Management and Budget, Executive Office of the President,
30 May.
Martin, S., Rice, N. and Smith, P.C. (2008) 'Does healthcare
spending improve health outcomes? Evidence from English
programme budgeting data', *Journal of Health Economics*, vol 27,
pp 826-42.
Mooney, G. and Lange, M. (1993) 'Antenatal screening: what
constitutes "benefit"?', *Social Science and Medicine*, vol 37,
pp 873-8.
Nord, E. (1999) *Cost-Value Analysis in Healthcare: Making Sense out
of QALYs*, Cambridge: Cambridge University Press.
Olsen, J.A. and Donaldson, C. (1998) 'Helicopters, hearts and
hips: using willingness to pay to set priorities for public sector
healthcare programmes', *Social Science and Medicine*, vol 46,
pp 1-12.
Parsonage, M. and Neuberger, H. (1992) 'Discounting and health
benefits', *Health Economics*, vol 1, pp 71-5.
Rawlins, M. and Culyer, A. (2004) 'National Institute for Clinical
Excellence and its value judgements', *British Medical Journal*,
vol 329, pp 224–27.
Shaw, J.W., Johnson, J.A. and Coombs, S.J. (2005) 'US valuation
of the EQ-5D health states: development and testing of the DI
model', *Medical Care*, vol 43, pp 203-20.
Torrance, G.W. (1986) 'Measurement of health state utilities for
economic appraisal: a review', *Journal of Health Economics*, vol 5,
pp 1-30.

SEVEN

What's your health worth?

Introduction

How can life and health be valued in monetary terms? Abhorrent though this may seem, life and health are evaluated in this way every day when decisions are made about what resources to allocate to health services, and within these services, how much to allocate to different programmes of care, and, even at the level of patient care, when decisions are made about who to treat, who not to treat or who has to wait. Two areas within the public sector that have made significant progress in developing evaluation methods are health and safety, especially transport safety. Environmental economics is also at the forefront of the development and application of evaluation methods. However, the strong links between health and safety with respect to their impact on life-saving and quality-of-life improvements make them a useful focus for this chapter.

The aims of the chapter, therefore, are to reflect current state-of-the-art in estimating monetary values for health and safety, and to suggest important next steps for research in these fields and how you as a reader may want to participate. The focus will initially be on health, because it is in this area that much recent debate has occurred about the need for monetary evaluation. It would seem natural then to move on to safety, this being an environment in which monetary evaluation appears to be acceptable up to a point (albeit still controversial). Lessons learned from experiences in these fields lead us to a discussion of the extent to which methods and results in one area can be brought together with those from the other and, indeed, more broadly across the public sector, so setting a research agenda as to how this might be achieved. Your participation would involve answering some of the weird and wonderful questions economists ask of people when conducting surveys aimed at putting a value on life or health.

Quality adjusted life years and willingness to pay

The issue of evaluating health in monetary terms has recently come to the fore internationally as a result of the creation of health technology assessment (HTA) agencies in several countries. In offering guidance to the health care systems in which they reside about the uptake (or maintenance) of health interventions, such agencies weigh up the costs and benefits involved. If it is thought necessary to express these costs and benefits in a common metric, usually money, the question raised is what value to place on improvements in length and quality of life. A similar situation arises when transport departments need to place a value on human life saved and non-fatal injuries avoided when considering road safety improvements that reduce the risk of accidents.

In England, when the National Institute for Health and Clinical Excellence (NICE) was first conceived, one of its aims, as stated by the UK House of Commons Health Committee in 2002, was 'to produce a common currency of effectiveness for the NHS'. The quality adjusted life year (QALY) has emerged as that common currency. There is a national 'tariff' for making quality adjustments to years of life, based on the five-dimensional generic health state classification system introduced in Chapter Six (see Box 6.1). The original aim of developing the QALY was to have a more complete measure of health gain than one based on survival alone and, with a more complete measure, to permit competing and quite disparate interventions to be compared on the basis of their cost per QALY gained. In most cases, the intervention with the lowest cost per QALY gained would be recommended for more resources at the expense of interventions with a relatively high cost per QALY gained. This reflects the dominant evaluation paradigm in health economics to date, whereby cost–utility analyses are conducted using the QALY as a measure of benefit.

However, returning to HTA agencies operating at the national level, many of the recommendations made by such organisations involve considerations of the costs and benefits of single interventions, where there is no comparison between alternatives. In such cases, the decisions about which intervention to provide are not obvious and the question concerns the value placed on QALY gains. This is further exacerbated by the challenges of considering aspects beyond the health effects captured by QALYs and how benefits produced by health care can be compared with those arising from investments in other areas of the public sector that are not (and often cannot be) valued in terms of QALYs. Hence, there is a need for a monetary measure to reflect the value of a QALY. The monetary measure that forms the basis of the review in this chapter is willingness to pay (WTP). One point to note in addition to the information provided in Chapter Six is the importance of distinguishing WTP, as a measure of benefit, from the cost of a good. Many people would be willing to pay more than the market-clearing price of a good. For individuals, the difference between benefit, as represented by their maximum WTP for the good, and the price paid by them for the good represents a gain in well-being from having the good provided.

The WTP method was first applied in the area of health in a well-known study by Acton in 1973 concerning heart attacks. There were relatively few subsequent studies in the area of health, probably as a result of the QALY being perceived as a more acceptable measure of benefit than one that valued life in monetary terms. Indeed, on the face of it, it would seem appear to be problematic to use WTP measures to inform decisions about the allocation of resources for commodities such as health care where such decisions are supposed to be made on the basis of (some notion of) need. This is because WTP is obviously associated with ability to pay. However, as noted in Chapter Six, my own work, with Steve Birch and Amiram Gafni of McMaster University (2002), has shown this need not impede the use of WTP in health care economic evaluations; whatever the method used to value benefits, including QALYs, it will suffer from the same distributional concerns. Since the early 1990s, WTP has taken off again, and, more recently and more relevant for this chapter, the two strands of literature have merged around the issue of WTP for a QALY.

Evaluating safety

The first empirical application of WTP (by Davis in 1963) was in the area of environmental policy evaluation. During the 1970s, the method was further developed in studies of the valuation of human life as applied to safety and transport policies. One of the classic papers on this subject is by the renowned Michael Jones-Lee and colleagues, published in 1985. Carried out over a 30-year period, this work has involved the development of methods to elicit a 'value of statistical life' and, thus, is closely related to the challenge of valuing a QALY (or 'healthy year').

Until the 1980s, most countries that explicitly addressed the public sector safety evaluation issue tended to use some variant of the so-called 'gross output' or 'human capital' approach. Under this approach, the primary component of the 'cost' of premature death is treated as the discounted present value of an individual's future output extinguished as a result of their premature demise. In some countries (including the UK), a further more-or-less arbitrary allowance was then added to the gross output figure to reflect the 'pain, grief and suffering' of victims and/or their surviving dependents and relatives. Values for the prevention of premature death are then defined in terms of the costs avoided.

To give an example of the costs and values that emerge under the gross output approach, the UK Department for Transport's most recent gross output figure, based on the value for the prevention of a road fatality and on national averages, was £180,330 in 1985 prices including a 28% allowance for pain, grief and suffering. Updated for inflation and growth of real output per capita, this figure would stand at some £500,000 in 2004 prices.

Not surprisingly, many economists have objected to the gross output approach on the grounds that most people almost certainly value safety largely because of their aversion to the prospect of their own and others' death and injury, rather than a concern to preserve current and future levels of output and income. It has therefore been argued that values of safety ought ideally to reflect people's 'pure' preferences for safety per se, rather than be defined in terms of effects on output and income, as in the gross output approach.

However, to define and estimate values of safety in this way clearly requires some means of measuring people's preferences for safety and, more particularly, their *strength* of preference. How can one do this? Arguably, the most natural measure of the extent of an individual's strength of preference for anything is the maximum amount they would be willing to pay for it. This amount reflects not only people's valuation of the desired good or service relative to other potential objects of expenditure, but also their varying *ability* to pay – which is itself a manifestation of society's overall resource constraint.

So, under what has naturally come to be known as the 'willingness to pay' approach to evaluating safety, one first seeks to establish the maximum amounts that those affected would individually be willing to pay for (typically small) improvements in their own and others' safety. These amounts are then simply aggregated across all individuals to arrive at an overall value for the safety improvement concerned. The resultant figure is thus a clear reflection of what the safety improvement is 'worth' to the affected group, relative to the alternative ways in which each individual might have spent his or her limited income. Furthermore, defining values of safety in this way effectively 'mimics' the operation of market forces – in circumstances in which markets typically do not exist – insofar as such forces can be seen as vehicles for allowing individual preferences to interact with relative scarcities and production possibilities to determine the allocation of a society's scarce resources.

In order to standardise values of safety that are derived from the WTP approach and render them comparable with values obtained under other approaches (such as gross output), the concept of the prevention of a 'statistical' fatality or injury is applied. To illustrate this concept, consider an example, devised by my colleague Phil Shackley, that we use in teaching medical students whereby we ask them to imagine they are going abroad for a period of study. This is provided in Box 7.1.

Imagine that 100,000 people were asked this question and they each were prepared to pay an additional £40. This would mean that they would collectively be willing to pay £4 million in order to save four lives. It is not known in advance who these four people would be, so the term used to describe them is 'statistical' fatalities.

Box 7.1: Willingness to pay for road safety improvement

Imagine that you have to make a long coach trip in a foreign country. You have been given £200 for your travel expenses and the name of a coach service that will take you to your destination for exactly £200. The risk of being killed on the coach journey with this firm is 8 in 100,000. You can choose to travel with a safer coach company if you want to, but the fare will be higher and you will have to pay the higher fare yourself.

How much extra, if anything, would you be prepared to pay to use a coach service with a risk of being killed of 4 in 100,000?

Dividing the aggregate WTP of £4 million by the expected number of fatalities avoided (four) would give what is referred to as a WTP-based *value of preventing one statistical fatality* (VPF) (or alternatively as the *value of statistical life* (VOSL)) of £1 million. The groundbreaking work of Michael Jones-Lee at Newcastle University (including his 1985 paper) has used more sophisticated versions of such questions to derive VPFs in many countries, as will be seen below.

Clearly, in the example above, the average individual WTP, of £40, for the average individual risk reduction of 4 in 100,000 is a reflection of the rate at which people in the group are willing to trade off wealth against risk 'at the margin', in the sense that the trade-offs typically involve small variations in wealth and small variations in risk. Empirical work on the valuation of safety thus tends to focus on these individual marginal wealth/risk trade-off rates.

On a somewhat more cautionary note, it is extremely important to appreciate that, defined in this way, the VPF is not a 'value (or price) of life' in the sense of a sum that any given individual would accept in compensation for the certainty of his or her own death – for most of us, no finite sum would suffice for this purpose, so that in this sense life is literally priceless. Rather, the VPF is aggregate WTP for typically very small reductions in individual risk of death (which, realistically, is what most safety improvements really offer at the individual level).

But how, in fact, are WTP values of safety estimated in practice? Broadly speaking, two variants of empirical estimation have been employed to derive WTP-based values of safety. These are known respectively as the 'revealed preference' (or 'implied value') and the 'contingent valuation' (or 'expressed value').

Basically, the revealed preference approach involves the identification of situations in which people actually do trade off income or wealth against physical risk – for example, in labour markets where riskier jobs can be expected to command clearly identifiable wage premia. The difficulty with the revealed preference approach when applied to labour market data is that it depends on being able to disentangle risk-related wage differentials from the many other factors that enter into the determination of wage rates. This approach also presupposes that workers are well informed about the risks they actually face in the workplace. In addition, those whose jobs do carry clearly identifiable wage premia for risk may not be representative of the workforce as a whole, in that such people almost certainly have a below-average degree of risk aversion.

The great advantage of the contingent valuation approach is that it allows the researcher to go directly and unambiguously to the relevant wealth/risk trade-off – at least, in principle, as in the hypothetical example in Box 7.1. On the other hand, the contingent valuation approach has the disadvantage of relying on the assumption that people are able to give considered, accurate and unbiased answers to hypothetical questions about typically small changes in already very small risks.

Turning to the question of the figures that are actually applied in practice, WTP-based values of safety are currently used in road project appraisal in the UK, US, Canada, Sweden and New Zealand, with several other countries employing values that have been substantially influenced by the results of WTP studies. More specifically, in the UK, the Department for Transport currently employs a figure of £1.4 million for the prevention of a statistical fatality in its roads project appraisal. This figure was based on the findings of a study that obtained estimates of the roads VPF using a variant of the contingent valuation approach – see Carthy and colleagues (1999). In the US, the Department of Transportation currently values the prevention of a statistical road fatality at $5 million, this being an update of a figure originally recommended in 1991 following a survey of the then-existing literature on empirical estimation of WTP-based values of safety.[1] In turn, Transport Canada applies a WTP-based value for the prevention of a statistical fatality of $Cdn 1.5 million in 1991 prices based on a survey of the literature. Updated for inflation and growth, this would be very close to the current UK value.

Finally, the WTP values used in Sweden and New Zealand were derived under the contingent valuation approach and in 1999 prices are SEK 14.30 million (roughly £1.07 million) and $NZ 2.5 million (roughly £820,000) respectively, although in the latter case it should be noted that the New Zealand Land Transport Safety Authority is considering increasing the figure to $NZ 4 million (roughly £1.32 million) on the basis of recommendations following an extensive recent contingent valuation study.

Recently, both quantitative and qualitative research has cast doubt on the reliability and validity of WTP values for safety derived through the direct contingent valuation method. As well as sequencing and framing effects, a prominent issue has been the lack of ability of the method to account for embedding and scope. That is, respondents tend to view safety improvements as a 'good thing' and, therefore, will often state much the same WTP for different sizes of risk reduction, whether for fatal or non-fatal injuries. It may be unreasonable to expect respondents to give accurate answers to hypothetical questions that involve direct trade-offs between wealth and small reductions in risk. Therefore, Carthy and colleagues (1999) suggested a less direct contingent valuation/standard gamble 'chained' approach that breaks down the valuation process into a series of more manageable steps that involve chaining together responses to WTP and standard gamble questions. A variant of this for use in valuing a QALY is shown below.

From life to QALYs

A straightforward way to combine work in health and safety valuation areas is to take the well-established roads VPF for the UK and, from it, attempt to model the value of a QALY. For example, if we take a representative death avoided as being that of a person aged 35, assume that the VPF is £1.4 million (or £1.4 × 10⁶) and that the person concerned would have lived for another 40 years, a rough calculation of the value of a life year gained by that person would be as follows:

$$V = \frac{£1.4 \times 10^6}{40} \tag{1}$$

$$= £35,000$$

Conveniently, V is close to the value of a QALY espoused by Rawlins and Culyer in their 2004 *British Medical Journal* paper referred to in Chapter 6. However, if one were to assume that not all of the 40 years gained would be spent in full health (especially later years) and a discount rate, whereby future years (and QALYs) are valued less than current ones, the denominator in (1) would fall, thus raising the value of a QALY above £35,000. For example, if the discount rate were taken to be 3.5%, the annualised sum that would have a discounted present value of £1.4 million over 40 years would be £77,300. In a recent paper with Helen Mason and Mike Jones-Lee (Mason et al, 2009), I looked at less simplistic ways of making this calculation, but I am sure you get the point. An important point to make is that this value is based on an original VPF gained by asking people about their WTP to avoid risk of death in a forthcoming time period (for example, the coming year). When estimating values based on questions about health gain scenarios that involve only quality-of-life improvements, with no extension to life, the values are substantially lower, at around £10,000 per QALY – again, see Mason et al (2009). So, it could be that life-saving QALYs are worth more than QALYs that improve health without actually saving lives or extending length of life. To many, this would make intuitive sense. This is why we rescue people stranded on mountainsides and why we do not switch off dialysis machines, neither of which is particularly attractive in terms of QALY gains for resources invested.

Survey research on the value of a QALY

In the medium term, it may be more prudent to move to an estimate of the value of a QALY based on actual survey research, in the same way that the VPF used in the safety field was derived. Everything we have discussed so far points to the need for such research to take place. Indeed, the Danes have already attempted this through the work of Dorte Gyrd-Hansen (2004).

But what might such a survey look like? There are two main approaches, albeit with several variants within each. The first, and more complex, is a version of the 'chained' approach referred to above. Here, you might first be given a description of a health state that would involve a degree of impairment compared with your current health. Let us say the heath state is for a stomach condition of the sort described in Box 7.2.

You might then be asked about whether you would be prepared to pay anything to avoid being in this state, and, if so, what is the maximum amount you are willing to pay. In the second part of the chain, you could be asked a standard gamble question of the sort shown in Figure 6.4 but this time with the health state in Box 7.2 inserted in place of 'being on dialysis' and portrayed as lasting for rest of life. In this gamble, one option would leave you with the stomach condition for certain and another involves a gamble with varying probabilities of dying immediately or returning to full health. Let us assume that, for you, the probability of return to full health at which you find it difficult to choose between the stomach condition for certain and taking the gamble is 0.95 and that your WTP to avoid a year in the stomach condition is £1,000. Dividing £1,000 by 0.05 (which comes from subtracting 0.95 from a value of full health of 1) would give you a QALY value of £20,000. This can be done across several individuals to arrive at an average value of a QALY for a population.

Such a scheme was devised by the eminent economist, Graham Loomes, as part of a recent research project in which we were members of the same project team. The scheme is highly innovative and, being new, demonstrated some challenges with people being unwilling to gamble in the standard gamble part of the procedure

---

Box 7.2: Stomach condition for rest of life

Initially you will have severe stomach pains, diarrhoea, vomiting and fever for seven days, severe enough to interfere with most of your usual activities.

Things then improve, but for the rest of your life you will suffer an episode of stomach discomfort and sickness every couple of weeks, with each episode lasting for two to three days. These episodes are not as severe, but may interfere with some of your usual activities.

and being willing to pay different amounts depending on the severity of scenarios presented to respondents. This is not new and indicates once more that there is more than one value of a QALY. Despite these challenges, by most reasonable ways of aggregating the data across respondents, a QALY value of around £20,000–£40,000 would not be wide of the mark.

Another approach is much more direct and involves considering whether it is possible to ask respondents to answer questions about their WTP to avoid health detriments that amount to approximately one QALY. For example, let us imagine you could think of health being measured on a scale of 0–100%, where 0 = dead and 100% = full health. Then, again assuming you are in full health, I might ask you what is the most you would be willing to pay to avoid a 10% drop in your health over the next 10 years, after which you would return to full health anyway. In QALY terms, a 10% loss for 10 years is equivalent to one QALY, so your answer would represent a particular QALY value. However, once again, there are several ways of asking this question: you could experience a 25% drop in health for four years or have one year of full health added on to your life. They will each result in different QALY values, so, again, there is no single answer. But, as with the explained method above, the potential has been shown to provide a range of answers that will be useful to decision makers, not only about how to allocate resources but also about what to spend on health care.

Various scenarios based on this second approach are shown in the Appendix to this book, where you will find a questionnaire. I invite you to answer the questions. The only problem with completing the questionnaire in this format is that it is assumed that you are 40 years of age and will live until you are 80. A more innovative form of the questionnaire is available online at http://research.ncl.ac.uk/eurovaq/ questionnaires.html. This version is more interactive, with questions based on your current stated age and your own estimate of what age you will live to, and so is a bit more realistic. As a continuation of the research project, we can gradually store up a databank of responses from interested members of the public. We can keep you informed of progress on resulting values among respondents at http://research. ncl.ac.uk/eurovaq/results.html.

Adjusting values for socially relevant concerns

It may also be important to adjust values to account for important theoretically relevant, informational and societal aspects that have been shown in health and other applied literatures to have an impact on values. These aspects include the information presented to respondents, age, health status (accounting for both quantity and quality of life), and broader societal factors such as age, initial health state (or severity), culpability and so on.

As far as the latter is concerned, it may be necessary to have different values of a QALY for different sets of circumstances. Indeed, in the case of safety, it has long been supposed that factors such as voluntariness, control, responsibility, catastrophe potential and so on – or to use a catch-all term 'dread' – may well lead to substantially different VPFs in different contexts. However, recent work by a team of colleagues at Newcastle University, led by Sue Chilton (2006), has found that, for a range of hazards involving risks of immediate death – such as road or rail accidents, fires in public places or drowning – significant differences in the degree of dread associated with such hazards by members of the public are largely offset by the fact that high dread hazards typically have lower levels of baseline risk, resulting in preference-based VPFs that do not differ greatly across the hazards concerned. So, in the UK, your life (based on aggregated valuations of small risk reductions) is still worth approximately £1.4 million according to the survey research.

Most of the research on QALYs has focused on whether health gains (usually QALYs) should be weighted differently according to the age of beneficiaries or the severity of their condition. Very few studies have applied actual weights elicited from members of the public to QALYs as such. However, an important question is whether health gain (however described) is allowed to vary across the choices (usually pairwise) faced by respondents. Many studies use a person trade-off method, ascribed originally to the work of Erik Nord. Using this method, you might be asked how many people of certain characteristics (for example, in terms of stage of life and/or severity of condition) achieving some sort of health (or QALY) gain would be judged equivalent to, say, 100 people with different characteristics who might also achieve such a gain. If the response is a number less than 100, it means that the gains to the former group are valued higher than those to the latter. Series of such questions can be asked to try to establish what these 'weights' would be for one individual and the responses aggregated to establish what the weights might be at the population level. There is a small but growing number of such studies. For those studies that show differences between groups, weights on health gains obtained by the most favoured over the least favoured group, across variables such as age and severity, can vary from 3:1 to 11:1. Generally, younger people (but not always the youngest) and those in severe health states (but not always the most severe) tend to be favoured over other groups.

Other studies, however, have shown that respondents do not wish to give preference to one group over another and that health gain is what counts. This would seem to fit with the positions of HTA agencies and health ministries around the world, none of which has adopted any explicit set of weightings. It would also seem to fit with the abandoned attempt by the US Environmental Protection Agency to instigate a 'senior health discount' on older lives saved, as mentioned in Chapter Six. The irony is that the weightings proposed come from surveys of members of the public. Is it the methods underlying the surveys that are wrong or is there something wrong with the HTA agencies and ministries that are not adopting the weightings? More work needs to be done in this area, but, for the moment, at least in England, it would seem that a year of healthy life (or a QALY) will remain at £20,000–£30,000. Do you agree? What do your own survey results say?

Conclusion

Now you know what governments think your life and your health is worth. But note that these assessments are based on surveys of the general public, so, they are, to some extent, an approximation of what you think.

The methods are developing, so it is important to know how you feel about the numbers they produce and the ways the values are derived. Do these numbers need to be more nuanced? Is a QALY gained through saving a life worth more than one gained from improving quality of life only? What about QALYs for children versus those at more advanced stages of life? What about people in more severe states? Is there anything else that should count?

Two other points are worth making at this stage. The reader may be thinking that all this can be achieved simply by asking people to rank services from most to least preferred until the health care budget is spent and/or by asking people how they would divide up the health care 'pie' across services. However, these methods do not tell us how strongly people feel, which can only be reflected in some notion of sacrifice. To an economist, something is not of value unless one is prepared to sacrifice something else in order to get it. In deriving QALYs, people are asked to sacrifice certainty (in the case of the standard gamble) or time (as in the case of the time trade-off). In this chapter, that sacrifice has been made in the form of money. This also has the advantage of providing a common unit of account, as, if people rank services differently or divide the pie differently, there is no recognised way to 'add up' these preferences to get an overall social judgement.

This leads to my second point, however. It might appear that basing the value of a life or a QALY on individual WTP values would result in higher values for the better-off and lower values for those on lower incomes. However, the point of asking a cross-section of the population about their WTP is not to differentiate between income groups but to obtain a value that takes proper account of society's overall budget constraint. Advocates of the WTP approach would tend to argue for one value, based on some measure of central tendency, to be applied to each member of society regardless of income. Indeed, public sector agencies that employ WTP-based values invariably apply the same *value*, based on the population *average*, to all income groups.

Despite appearances to the contrary, there is still much work to be done in developing such economics-based methods for valuing outputs for the whole public sector, not just for health care. The challenges outlined in this chapter are immense, but so also has been the progress described. In the context of safety, the values that exist are now routinely used in policy making in the UK, Canada, New Zealand, Sweden and the US. This research work, essentially addressing the fundamental issue of the 'value of life', has the rare distinction in social and management research of being both groundbreaking and having fed directly into policy. Extension and replication of the work in the health field has the potential to be equally profound in terms of scientific quality and use in policy, and, if successful, may lead to further endeavours across the public sector. If more accurate estimates of the value of life and health can be obtained, resource allocation decisions that follow from their application will also be more efficient, leading to better health and more lives saved. What could be more important than that?

Note

[1] The US figure is higher than that in other countries because it is derived from what are known as 'revealed-preference' labour market data, in which workers essentially reveal a wage premium they are willing to accept for being employed in a riskier occupation. Traditionally, willingness-to-accept values associated with risk increases are higher than WTP values for corresponding risk reductions. This is one possible explanation, of course, the others being that income per capita and general attitudes to physical risk are different in the US compared with elsewhere.

Further reading

Acton, J.P. (1973) *Evaluating Public Programs to Save Lives: The Case of Heart Attacks*, Report No R950RC, Santa Monica, CA: RAND Corporation.

Baker, R., Bateman, I., Donaldson, C., Jones-Lee, M., Lancsar, E., Loomes, G., Mason, H., Odejar, M., Pinto Prades, J.L., Robinson, A., Ryan, M., Shackley, P., Smith, R., Sugden, R. and Wildman, J. (2010) 'Weighting and valuing quality adjusted life years using stated preference methods: preliminary results from the social value of a QALY project', *Health Technology Assessment*, vol 14, no 27.

Carthy, T., Chilton, S., Covey, J., Hopkins, L., Jones-Lee, M., Loomes, G., Pidgeon, N. and Spencer, A. (1999) 'On the contingent valuation of safety and the safety of contingent valuation: part 2 – the CV/SG "chained" approach', *Journal of Risk and Uncertainty*, vol 17, pp 187-213.

Chilton, S.M., Jones-Lee, M. and Metcalf, H. (2006) 'Dread risks', *Journal of Risk and Uncertainty*, vol 33, pp 165–82.

Davis, R.K. (1963) 'Recreation planning as an economic problem', *Natural Resources Journal*, vol 3, pp 239-49.

Donaldson, C. (1999) 'Valuing the benefits of publicly provided healthcare: does "ability to pay" preclude the use of "willingness to pay"?', *Social Science and Medicine*, vol 49, pp 551-63.

Donaldson, C., Birch, S. and Gafni, A. (2002) 'The pervasiveness of the "distribution problem" in economic evaluation in healthcare', *Health Economics*, vol 11, pp 55-70.

Gyrd-Hansen, D. (2004) 'Willingness to pay for a QALY', *Health Economics*, vol 12, pp 1049-60.

Jones-Lee, M.W., Hammerton, M. and Philips, P.R. (1985) 'The value of safety: results of a national sample survey', *Economic Journal*, vol 95, pp 49-72.

Mason, H., Jones-Lee, M.W. and Donaldson, C. (2009) 'Modelling the monetary value of a QALY: a new approach based on UK data', *Health Economics*, vol 18, pp 933-50.

Nord, E. (1999) *Cost-Value Analysis in Healthcare: Making Sense out of QALYs*, Cambridge: Cambridge University Press.

EIGHT

Conclusion

We started by describing public funded health care as a series of quid pro quos; in other words, a set of compromises. Knowing what we now know, what compromises are left to make? Is it time to draw some lines in the sand?

It's official: publicly funded health care provides 'competitive advantage'

First, we know we can argue strongly that the public funding of health care is both equitable and efficient. Governments need to be explicit about this and support such a position. For example, and the reason I say 'it's official', the Canadian government, on its Health Canada website, is very explicit about the gains the Canadian economy derives from its publicly funded health care system:

> The competitive advantage that publicly financed healthcare provides to Canadian business is significant. Public financing spreads the cost of providing health services equitably across the country. In addition, financing health insurance through the taxation system is cost-efficient because it does not require a separate collection process.

More governments should stand behind their health care system in this way.

What role for health care reforms?

Within the general policy area of health care reform, little or no faith can be placed in changes aimed at pushing the burden of health care decision making on to patients and the public. For example, financial incentives in the form of user charges do not work, whether assessed in terms of cost containment, efficiency or equity. The same applies to medical savings accounts and, to a lesser extent, patient budgets. Naïve politicians, other policy makers, doctors and even economists will 'rediscover' user charges and the like from time to time. We need to keep shooting down their arguments.

What of other reforms? Here, context is everything. Internal markets within publicly funded systems do seem to have had some positive impact. However, such reforms are never left in place long enough for us to be definitive, and, with efficiency being merely one goal of health care, any discernible impact has been small. Moreover, such reforms have not been able to arrest the continued slide into an acute-sector-dominated form of medicine. This model is outdated. We need to get away from the view that we are fit one minute, seriously ill the next, miraculously treated, and thus returned to full health. Societies are now dealing with frailty in old age, learning disabilities, mental health, alcohol and drug dependence, chronic disease, dementia and so on. But incentive systems and resulting care plans are just not geared up for this, serving neither efficiency nor equity and perpetuating our failings in public health. Giving responsibility for budgets to those closer to patients but outside of the hospital system, such as general practitioners in the UK context, may help achieve the required practice change. Such incentives can be combined with others through 'blended payment systems'. The idea here is that, depending on objectives, different payment systems will have different degrees of success. In addition to budgeting as a way of encouraging the trade off between cost and quality, a fee per item of service system (for things we want doctors to do a lot of) and salaries (maybe for hospital doctors, whom we wish to be well paid but without reward explicitly tied to volume of activity) each have a place. The key is to decide on the objectives.

In the US, the very basics of competition (freedom and tailoring of insurance packages to risk) so cherished by its citizens actually result in health care reforms failing to achieve the desired goals (of maintaining quality and keeping costs down). Ironically, a restricted type of competition, where consumers are locked into the broader system and cannot opt in and out and the competitive element applies mainly to the supply side, may work better. Americans still need to grasp this notion, and, when they do, the more privileged members of US society will see that they are not losing much at all, if anything.

A challenge for all systems is to ensure that physician behaviour is harnessed so as to best serve the notions of value and efficiency for patients and the population. Clinicians are best placed, especially if they are budget-holders, to deliver the care plans that best meet the needs of patients and serve the system efficiency. Some countries have more work to do on this than others. The challenge for public systems is to strengthen the purchasing function so as to allow these purchasers (who could be family doctors) to move resources around the system more in line with best care to meet population need within resource limitations.

Structurally, one way of aiding purchasers might be to have health technology assessment agencies, such as the National Institute for Health and Clinical Excellence (NICE) in England, work more closely with them, which may even involve the NICE agenda being set by primary care trusts (PCTs) or their equivalent. After all, NICE and PCTs are the only two entities in the NHS in England that represent geographically defined populations. Although processes may need to be in place to ensure timely assessment of new drugs and other technologies coming on to the market, why should NICE and PCTs not be working more in line with each other in a parallel process to systematically eradicate unwarranted variations in provision of care across the country and to disinvest from unproductive services (that is, those producing no benefit at all and those producing only small gains for the resources invested)?

From culture of contentment to culture of containment

Apart from these suggested changes, reform is unlikely to get us very far, amounting to the health care equivalent of fiddling while Rome burns. Continued reform (or fiddling) allows politicians to avoid the real issue of setting priorities in a more explicit way so as to sustain our publicly funded systems (stopping Rome burning). The basic problem is that, in the public sectors of many economies, a culture of contentment has arisen over the past two decades. No one has had to worry about managing scarcity in the good times, and thus the skills for doing so in the bad times are simply not there.

The key now is to rebuild these skills and, with that, change the culture. This can only be done through education and by providing support to those making the tough decisions. It is a major indictment of our managerial and clinical educational systems that professionals are not routinely taught health economics, the 'science of scarcity', when they have to manage scarce resources on a day-to-day basis. Likewise, education should focus not on the latest management fads typically taught on postgraduate business administration programmes but rather on research methods that will help managers articulate what a health outcome is and be able to appraise evidence on whether outcomes are improved by new ways of doing things. Such an educational change would create an 'enquiring and open' as opposed to a 'fixing and closed' culture in health care management.

In terms of providing support, regional priority-setting units should be created across countries to develop and support the implementation of frameworks to deal with the economic, ethical and legal issues that need to be addressed constantly in order to set priorities. Legislative trends in many countries will require decision makers to have robust processes behind the decisions they make, especially when restricting access, and they will also have to be able to deal equitably with the growing number of people who claim to be exceptional and, therefore, worthy of special treatment. Such units should develop processes that help local decision makers seek out waste (for example, through unnecessary variations in health care delivery) and impose standard working. But such 'lean thinking' is only part of the wider framework. Of course, we should be lean before we consider genuine cutbacks in effective services. However, if the rumours are to be believed and some countries are required to make savings of up to 20% on health budgets, we will have to think beyond lean. In addition to achieving such 'technical' efficiencies, frameworks will be required to help deal with difficult situations whereby effective care may have to be withdrawn from one group so that another can benefit. The only framework that encompasses all of these issues (including 'lean') is programme budgeting and marginal analysis.

Ethically, clinicians should be familiar with the economic evidence for the different possible procedures in their area of care and should act on this evidence in order to stop inefficient practices and enhance efficient ones, so maximising benefit from their limited budgets. This is the clinical equivalent of 'getting your house in order' before coming to ask for more resources. As with many good ideas that still have not been taken up in health care, this was the very approach advocated by Florence Nightingale, who, when asked how she might make use of a fund collected in her name by the British public during the 1850s, replied: 'If I had a plan, it would be simply to take the poorest and least organised hospital in London and, putting myself there, to see what I could do – not touching the Fund for years, until experience had shown how the Fund might best be available' (cited in Small, 1999, pp 67-8).

Thus, as well as advocating other sensible approaches to health care management, such as routine collection data on health outcomes, Florence Nightingale was a pioneer of health economics, even supporting the use of programme budgeting and marginal analysis.

Such an approach requires that clinicians and managers become familiar with methods of economic evaluation, enhancing their ability to appraise the economic evidence. Where the evidence does not exist, they need to lead research proposals with health economists and other methodologists in order to generate it. Currently, clinicians tend to venture into science by donning another white coat, of the sort worn in a laboratory. The whole notion of the clinician-scientist needs to be recast, with clinicians thinking less about discovering some miracle cure and more about how to assess the outcome and efficiency of what they currently do and of new treatments. Furthermore, there are vast gains to be had in applying what we already know from research than in so-called 'discovery' research. Clinicians should therefore be participating in research on how to change the behaviour of their own profession.

Ultimately moving away from the culture of contentment in health care resource allocation will make it more explicit that we need to consider fundamental issues of the value of life and health in society more widely. This can be done only by researchers, managers, clinicians, patients and the public working together to consider and define what is important, but recognising that not all can be provided and that there are limits, the consequence of which is that values have to be placed on what has been defined as important. Thus more research is required to address questions such as whether health gains achieved through saving life are worth more than gains from improving quality of life only. What about health gains for children versus those at more advanced stages of life? What about people in more severe states? Is a small life extension for those in terminal stages of cancer really worthwhile, given how else those resources could be used? Is there anything else that should count? We need to be able to put numbers on these things; both public and government need to accept that, and the research community needs to be able to deliver it.

With a questioning public, enquiring patients, curious physicians and sceptical managers, all recognising scarcity and having open discussions about how to manage it, not only will publicly funded health care be sustainable, but also resources will be used to best serve the interests of the community. This will be crucial during the forthcoming period of public sector austerity. However, its longer-lasting impact will be that we will have a generation of professionals who know how to manage scarce resources, which is just as ethical an endeavour when public services are relatively well funded as when we have credit crunch health care. As health economics pioneer Alan Williams (1987) might have said, this would indeed be a cheerful outcome of applying the 'dismal science'.

Further reading

Small, H. (1999) *Florence Nightingale, Avenging Angel*, Constable: London.
Williams, A. (1987) 'Health economics: the cheerful face of a dismal science', in A. Williams (ed) *Health and Economics*, Macmillan: London.

Appendix:
'What's your health worth?'
A questionnaire

Governments around the world are always having to think about how much to spend on the health of their population and what priority to place on different ways of improving health.

One way of helping them to do this is to ask members of the public about how much they personally value different types of health improvement.

This is what we want to do with you in this questionnaire. Imagine that your health service is as efficient as it can be and that to buy 'extra health' you would have to pay out of your own pocket; you can even think of this as some form of taxation if you wish.

In this version of the questionnaire, we will ask you to make some assumptions about your age (you are a 40-year-old) and how long you might live, and also to assume you are in full health. In the online version of the questionnaire, we ask you to state your actual age, estimate how long you will live and to rate your health status and we then base the questions on these responses. So, the questions in the online form are tailored to you and are thus more realistic.

What follows is the slightly less realistic form of the questionnaire. On average, most people can expect to live for 80 years.

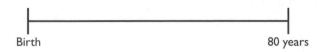

Birth   80 years

If we equate 0 with 'being dead' and 1 to being in 'full health', if people were to live each of these 80 years in the best of health for all ages, we would expect your 80 years to look like this:

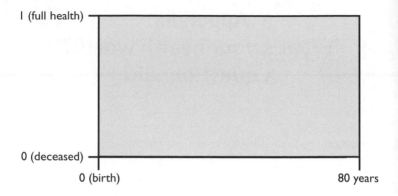

For you, as a 40-year-old, this would mean that, if you live the rest of your life in full health, your remaining 40 years would look like this:

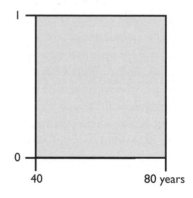

1. Now, imagine that, in one year's time, rather than living the next four years in full health, you will experience an illness that reduces your health to 75% (or 0.75) of full health, after which you will return to full health for the remaining years of your life. This is illustrated in this next diagram, where your 'loss' in health is shown by the dark-shaded area.

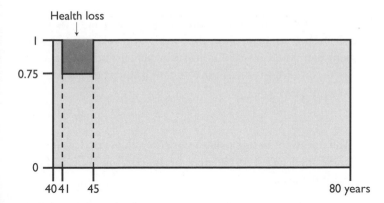

What would be your maximum willingness to pay to avoid this illness? (You can think about this as a one-off, lump-sum payment that you can make from your current income or savings or take out in a longer-term, interest-free loan to be paid back over a number of years.)

£ —————

2.   Now, imagine that you would experience the same reduction in your health for four years, but later in your life, at age 70. So, at that point, you will experience an illness that reduces your health to 75% (or 0.75) of full health for four years, after which you will return to full health for the remaining years of your life. This is illustrated in this next diagram, where, again, your 'loss' in health is shown by the dark-shaded area.

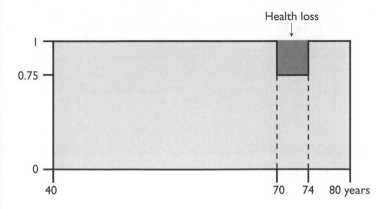

What would be your maximum willingness to pay to avoid this illness? (Again, you can think about this as a one-off, lump-sum payment that you can make from your current income or savings or take out in a longer-term, interest-free loan to be paid back over a number of years.)

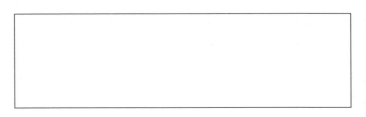

£ _____

3. You may want to think about why the values you have given in questions 1 and 2 are different or, indeed, the same, and make some notes here.

4. Now, imagine that, in one year's time, instead of facing the certainty of living for the next four years in 75% (or 0.75) of full health, you face a 10% chance of this happening. This is illustrated in the next diagram, where your 'loss' in health is again shown by the dark-shaded area, but with only a 10% chance of this loss occurring.

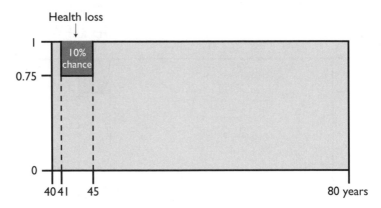

What would be your maximum willingness to pay to reduce the chance of having this illness from 10% to 0%. (You can think about this as a one-off, lump-sum payment that you can make from your current income or savings or take out in a longer-term, interest-free loan to be paid back over a number of years.

£

5. Now, imagine that, rather than living the next 10 years in full health, you will experience an illness that reduces your health to 90% (or 0.90) of full health, after which you will return to full health for the remaining years of your life. This is illustrated in this next diagram, where your 'loss' in health is shown by the dark-shaded area.

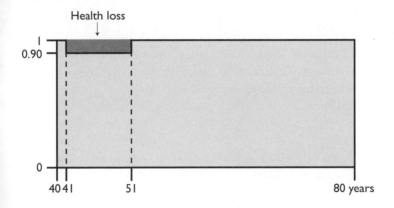

What would be your maximum willingness to pay to avoid this illness? (You can think about this as a one-off, lump-sum payment that you can make from your current income or savings or take out in a longer-term, interest-free loan to be paid back over a number of years.)

£

6. Now, imagine that you will experience the same reduction in your health for 10 years, but later in your life, at age 70. So, at that point, you will experience an illness that reduces your health to 90% (or 0.90) of full health for the last 10 years of your life.

This is illustrated in this next diagram, where, again, your 'loss' in health is shown by the dark-shaded area.

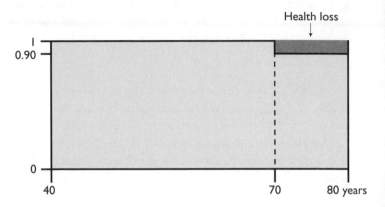

What would be your maximum willingness to pay to avoid this illness? (You can think about this as a one-off, lump-sum payment that you can make from your current income or savings or take out in a longer-term, interest-free loan to be paid back over a number of years.)

£ _____

7. Again, you may want to think about why the values you have given in questions 5 and 6 are different or, indeed, the same, and make some notes here. Also, you may want to think about your answers to 1 and 2 relative to 5 and 6.

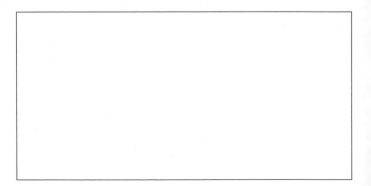

8. Now, imagine that, in one year's time, instead of facing the certainty of living for the next four years in 90% (or 0.90) of full health, you face a 10% chance of this happening. This is illustrated in the next diagram, where your 'loss' is again shown by the dark-shaded area, but with only a 10% chance of this loss occurring.

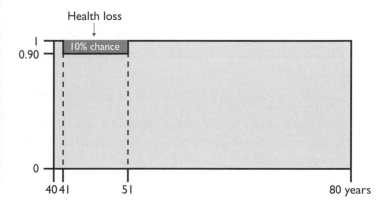

What would be your maximum willingness to pay to reduce the chance of having this illness from 10% to 0%? (You can think about this as a one-off, lump-sum payment that you can make from your current income or savings or take out in a longer-term, interest-free loan to be paid back over a number of years.)

£

9. Now, imagine that you can expect to live until you are 80 years old. At your current age, you are informed by a public health campaign/local doctors/primary care trust (PCT) that there is now a new treatment available that would reduce your chances of dying in any given year by a very small amount, resulting in your average life expectancy being increased by one year. You would spend this extra year in full health for someone of that age. This is illustrated in this next diagram, where, this time, your 'gain' in health is shown by the dark-shaded area.

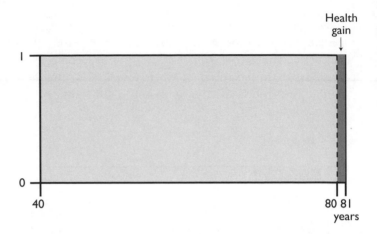

The treatment would involve taking one tablet at your current age. It is perfectly safe and has no harmful side effects. During the time between your current age and age 80, no better treatment will be developed.

What would be your maximum willingness to pay for this treatment? (You can think about this as a one–off, lump-sum payment that you can make from your current income or savings or take out a longer-term, interest-free loan to be paid back over a number of years).

£

10. Now, imagine that you can still expect to live until you are 80 years old. At your current age, you are informed by a doctor that you have a condition that will shorten your life by one year and there is now a new treatment available that would result in you being able to avoid this loss and restore your life expectancy to 80 (from 79) years. You would spend this 'extra' year in full health for someone of that age. Again, this is illustrated in this next diagram where your 'gain' in health is shown by the dark-shaded area.

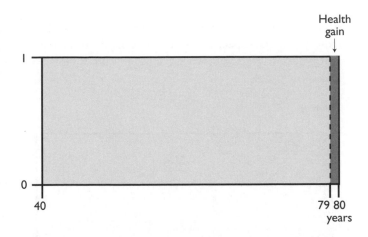

The treatment would involve taking one tablet at your current age. It is perfectly safe and has no harmful side effects. During the time between your current age and age 79, no better treatment will be developed.

What would be your maximum willingness to pay for this treatment? (You can think about this as a one-off, lump-sum payment that you can make from your current income or savings or take out a longer-term, interest-free loan to be paid back over a number of years).

£

11. In the last question, the gain in health comes a long way in the future. To try to think about getting this gain in the near future, and imagine now that you are in full health (or your current health state if not full health) but that you visit your doctor for a minor health complaint where he informs you that you have developed a condition that will cause you to slip into a coma for the next year. During this coma, you will feel no pain or sensation; it would be like being in a deep, peaceful sleep for a year (more than a year if not in full health). Before you went into the coma you would have time to make preparations for this year. After the year, you would wake up and regain full health (or health state prior to coma). All other aspects of your life would be unaffected during and after this year and you would

be able to pick up where you left off. However, it essentially reduces your life expectancy by one year. Again, this is illustrated in this next diagram, where your 'loss' in health is shown by the dark-shaded area.

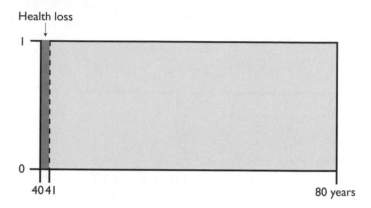

What would be your maximum willingness to pay to avoid this illness? (You can think about this as a one-off, lump-sum payment that you can make from your current income or savings or take out in a longer-term, interest-free loan to be paid back over a number of years.)

£

12. Again, you may want to think about why the values you have given in questions 9-11 are different or, indeed, the same, and make some notes here.

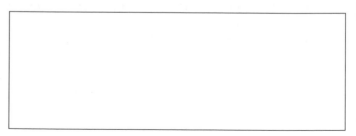

13. Now, imagine that you are currently in full health and that you are diagnosed with an illness that is terminal if untreated. Death from this illness would occur within a few months of the diagnosis if treatment is not received. A new treatment becomes available that could give you an extra year in full health. Again, this is illustrated in this next diagram, where your 'gain' in health is shown by the dark-shaded area.

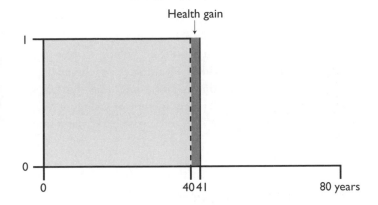

What would be the maximum amount you would be willing to pay for this treatment? (You can think about this as a one-off, lump-sum payment that you can make from your current income or savings or take out in a longer-term, interest-free loan to be paid back over a number of years.)

£ _____

14. Now, imagine that you are involved in an accident in which you sustain injuries that could prove fatal if not treated by emergency services within 10 minutes of the accident occurring. The standard response time is 20 minutes, which would lead to 1 in 100 patients dying before emergency services arrived, so a service that arrived within 10 minutes would eliminate that risk. If you survived, you would make a full recovery, return to full health and live to 80 years of age. This is illustrated in the next diagram by the dark-shaded area, but with only a 1% (1 in 100) chance of this loss occurring.

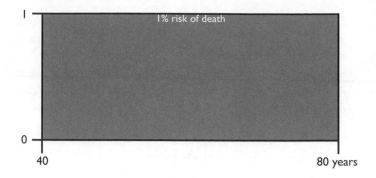

What is the maximum you would be willing to pay to have emergency services arrive within 10 minutes, so eliminating the risk? (You can think about this as a one-off, lump-sum payment that you can make from your current income or savings or take out in a longer-term, interest-free loan to be paid back over a number of years.)

£ ————

My thoughts on the responses

There are lots of problems with these types of question, but largely they have been included to get you thinking.

Q1-Q4

This is the simplest way of expressing a 1-QALY loss to people, by having a percentage drop in health (in this case 25%) for a fixed amount of time (four years), so that is why we started with these types of question.

Generally, because of time preference, people will give a higher willingness to pay to avoid the health (or QALY) loss in Q1 than in Q2. The impact is sooner in Q1, hence the higher values. But note that this is not the case for everyone. There will be some people who think they would rather be healthy when they are older or something like that and would state a greater willingness to pay in Q2. There are no right or wrong answers here.

All Q3 does is to try to bring in a bit of realism with respect to uncertainty of experiencing such a condition. Again, the willingness to pay should be less than in Q1, but the answer you give would be multiplied by 10 (because of the 10% risk) to arrive at a value of a QALY (that could be larger or smaller than in Q1 and Q2 depending on what your willingness to pay was, but in most cases it will be larger after multiplying by 10).

Q5-Q8

My comments here are essentially the same in terms of how you would compare these answers with each other. Here, the only difference to Q1-Q4 is that the 1-QALY loss is through a 10% drop for 10 years. QALY theorists would say your set of answers should be the same as for Q1-Q4, but you may think differently depending on what you think about a 10% loss or living with something for 10 years.

Q9-Q12

Here, we are trying to introduce the notion of gaining a QALY through extension to your life rather than improving quality of life. You may think intuitively that adding years to your survival would be seen as more important than adding to quality of life. However, the only way of expressing that is through giving you a small amount of time at the end of your life, which is what Q9 and Q10 are about. However, because these gains are so far in the future for most people, they tend to state quite a low willingness to pay for them (unless they are 70 years of age, of course). This is why we have introduced the rather unusual coma scenario in Q11 – to bring forward in time the idea of losing a year of life. No doubt this raised all sorts of other considerations in your mind, even though we tried to say that very little would be affected by this happening to you. Generally, people would state greater willingness to pay to avoid the QALY lost through the coma.

Q13 and Q14

These questions are introduced to give you different life-saving (as opposed to life-extending) scenarios. One is for a situation where life will be short anyway (because you have, for example, an illness such as terminal cancer) and the other for emergency services. The former is interesting as it leads to split opinions, with some people giving higher values just to keep living and because, if they are going to die anyway, they might as well spend what they have, and others reasoning that 'when you gotta go, you gotta go' or thinking of leaving a legacy for relatives (or others), thus giving quite low (or even zero) values. The value of a QALY that results from questions like Q14 tends to be relatively high.

Index

Note: The letter 't' following a page number indicates a table.

V

W